Basic Ophthalmology

for Medical Students and Primary Care Residents

Seventh Edition

Cynthia A. Bradford, MD

Executive Editor

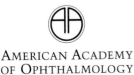

AMERICAN ACADEMY
OF OPHTHALMOLOGY

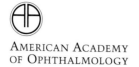

AMERICAN ACADEMY
OF OPHTHALMOLOGY

P.O. Box 7424
San Francisco, CA 94120-7424

Clinical Education Secretaries

Thomas A. Weingeist, PhD, MD
Senior Secretary for Clinical Education

Thomas J. Liesegang, MD
Secretary for Instruction

For the 7th Edition

Cynthia A. Bradford, MD, *Executive Editor*

Denise R. Chamblee, MD, *Revision Contributor*

Jennie M. Hunnewell, MD, *Revision Contributor*

Rebecca K. Morgan, MD, *Revision Contributor*

Scott C. Sigler, MD, *Revision Contributor*

Interspecialty Education Committee

Anne L. Coleman, MD, *Chair*

Terry J. Bergstrom, MD

Cynthia A. Bradford, MD

Deborah S. Jacobs, MD

Robert Jay Granadier, MD

Academy Clinical Education Staff

Kathryn A. Hecht, EdD
Vice President

Hal Straus
Director of Publications

William J. Hering, PhD
Director of Programs

Kevin Stepelton
Program Manager

Margaret Petela
Managing Editor

Ruth Modric
Production Manager

Beth T. Berkelhammer
Production Editor

Each author states that he or she has no significant financial interest or other relationship with the manufacturer of any commercial product mentioned in the text that he or she contributed to this publication or with the manufacturer of any competing commercial product.

Library of Congress Cataloging-in-Publication Data
Basic ophthalmology for medical students and primary
 care residents. — 7th ed. / Cynthia A. Bradford,
 executive editor.
 p.   cm.
 Includes bibliographical references and index.
 ISBN 1-56055-098-8 (pbk.)
 1. Ophthalmology.   2. Primary care (Medicine)
I. Bradford, Cynthia A., 1958–   .
 [DNLM: 1. Eye Diseases. 2. Diagnostic Techniques,
Ophthalmological. WW 100B3114 1999]
RE46.065 1999
617.7—dc21
DNLM/DLC   98-27992
 for Library of Congress   CIP

97 96 95 94   5 4 3 2 1

Contents

Chapter 6

Amblyopia and Strabismus   94

Chapter 7

Neuro-Ophthalmology   110

Chapter 8

Ocular Manifestations of Systemic Disease   129

Figures and Slides

Slides

Numbers for the color photos designated "Slide" in the text correspond to numbered slides in the companion *Basic Ophthalmology* Slide Set.

Preface

Basic Ophthalmology for Medical Students and Primary Care Residents is designed to help the user learn the techniques of a complete eye examination and the most important concepts of diagnosis and management of ocular disorders. The history of this textbook began in 1975 with the publication by the American Academy of Ophthalmology of a study guide in outline form for medical students. The book's developers identified seven common problem areas in ophthalmology and developed study objectives. Each subsequent edition was changed based on suggestions from users. The fifth edition, which was developed by the joint committee of the American Academy of Ophthalmology and the Association of University Professors of Ophthalmology, abandoned the outline form for chapters with expository text. The sixth edition, published in 1993, was one of the American Academy of Ophthalmology's most popular clinical education products, with 25,000 copies sold since its introduction. This seventh edition is an update of the excellent work of Dr. Frank Berson and the Medical Student Education Committee in response to recent changes in clinical medicine and health-care delivery, which have increased the need for primary care physicians-in-training in the areas of diagnosis, management, and referral of ocular disease.

Prior to undertaking this revision, a user evaluation of the sixth edition was conducted among previous authors, Academy members involved in medical student education, medical students, and primary care residents. Chapters have been revised based on the resulting recommendations. Much information and many photographs have been improved and updated. For example, glaucoma care has undergone significant changes in the past 5 years, and these are reflected in this edition's descriptions of glaucoma medications and tonometry.

As in previous editions, the seventh edition features a number of new photographs and updated and expanded annotated resources. The book's color photographs depicting normal and abnormal eye conditions are also available as a companion set of 78 color slides. Where appropriate, tables are presented to summarize textual information and facilitate study.

This book can be used in a variety of teaching settings. The concise presentation of information makes it ideal for brief ophthalmology rotations. If greater time is available, the resources can be consulted for more detail. Thus, the book is intended to be a flexible instrument that summarizes the important concepts, techniques, and facts of ophthalmology for all physicians, especially those in primary care. The Interspecialty Education Committee anticipates that medical students will use this book in conjunction with the comprehensive texts and other related resources annotated at the end of each chapter.

The current contributors would like to thank their predecessors on the Medical Student Education Committee who, partially through this book, built a great foundation for medical student learning. Current contributors include Denise R. Chamblee, MD; Jennie M. Hunnewell, MD; Rebecca K. Morgan, MD; and Scott C. Sigler, MD. Thanks are due the following individuals who contributed photographs to this edition: David W. Parke II, MD; Bradley K. Farris, MD; Reagan H. Bradford, Jr, MD; Anne L. Coleman, MD, PhD; and Neil R. Miller, MD.

Who's Who in Eye Care

Ophthalmologist

An ophthalmologist is a physician (doctor of medicine or doctor of osteopathy) who specializes in the medical and surgical care of the eyes and visual system and in the prevention of eye disease and injury. The ophthalmologist has completed four or more years of college premedical education, four or more years of medical school, one year of internship, and three or more years of specialized medical, surgical, and refractive training and experience in eye care. The ophthalmologist is a specialist who is qualified by lengthy medical education, training, and experience to diagnose, treat, and manage all eye and visual system problems and is licensed by a state regulatory board to practice medicine and surgery. The ophthalmologist is the medically trained specialist who can deliver total eye care: primary, secondary, and tertiary care services (ie, vision services, spectacles, contact lenses, eye examinations, medical eye care, and surgical eye care), diagnose general diseases of the body, and treat ocular manifestations of systemic diseases.

Optometrist

An optometrist is a health service provider who is involved exclusively with vision problems. Optometrists are specifically educated and trained by an accredited optometry college in a four-year course, but they do not attend medical school. They are state licensed to examine the eyes and to determine the presence of vision problems. Optometrists determine visual acuity and prescribe spectacles, contact lenses, and eye exercises. Optometrists may perform all services listed under the definition of opticians. Most states have passed legislation that permits optometrists to treat some eye conditions.

Optician

An optician is a professional who makes, verifies, delivers, and fits lenses, frames, and other specially fabricated optical devices and/or contact lenses upon prescription to the intended wearer. The optician's functions include prescription analysis and interpretation; determination of the lens forms best suited to the wearer's needs; the preparation and delivery of work orders for the grinding of lenses and the fabrication of eye wear; the verification of the finished ophthalmic products; and the adjustment, replacement, repair, and reproduction of previously prepared ophthalmic lenses, frames, and other specially fabricated ophthalmic devices.

Test Your Knowledge

Test your present awareness about eye care by taking this quick true-false quiz. The test contains many statements that you may have heard before. Answers follow.

1. Reading for prolonged periods in dim light can be harmful to the eyes.   T   F

2. Children should be taught not to hold their books too close when reading, because doing so can harm their eyes.   T   F

3. Wearing glasses that are too strong can damage the eyes.   T   F

4. If children sit too close to the television set, they may damage their eyes.   T   F

5. Older people who may be having trouble seeing should not use their eyes too much because they can wear them out sooner.   T   F

6. People with weak eyes should rest their eyes often to strengthen them.   T   F

7. In time, children usually outgrow crossed eyes.   T   F

8. Contact lenses can correct nearsightedness, so that eventually neither contact lenses nor eyeglasses will be needed.   T   F

9. Children who have a problem learning to read are likely to have an eye coordination problem and can be helped with special exercises.   T   F

10. A cataract can sometimes grow back after cataract surgery.   T   F

11. A cataract has to be "ripe" before surgery can be done.   T   F

12. Nearsighted people become farsighted as they age, and farsighted people become nearsighted.   T   F

13. In older people, a sign of healthy eyes is the ability to read the newspaper without glasses.   T   F

14. People who wear glasses should have their vision checked every year to determine whether a change in prescription is needed.   T   F

15. Watching a bright television picture in a dimly lighted room can be harmful to the eyes if done for long periods.   T   F

16. Ideally, all people should use an eyewash regularly to cleanse their eyes.   T   F

17. A blue eye should not be selected for transplantation into a brown-eyed person.   T   F

18. In rare instances, a contact lens can be lost behind the eye and even work its way into the brain.   T   F

19. A cataract is actually a film over the eye that can be peeled off with surgery.   T   F

20. Headaches are usually due to eye strain.   T   F

Answers

1. False. Except in extreme circumstances, the *way* in which light enters the eye is not important. Reading in dim light does not harm the eyes any more than taking a photograph in dim light would harm a camera.

2. False. Holding books close to the eyes to read is common in children, and no harm can come of it. Their eyes can accommodate (focus on near objects) easily and can keep near objects in sharp focus. In rare cases, holding a book close could be a sign of severe nearsightedness, which should be investigated; however, the habit of close reading itself will not cause nearsightedness in children.

3. False. Because glasses are hung in front of the eyes (from the nose and ears), they affect light, not the eye. Looking through them cannot harm the eyes. However, an incorrect prescription may result in blurred vision, which is uncomfortable and may lead to headaches.

4. False. Children with normal sight commonly want to sit close to the television set, just as they want to get close to reading material. This will not harm their eyes. All individuals will hold reading material or watch television at a distance that is comfortable for them.

5. False. The eyes are made for seeing. No evidence exists that using them for their purpose will wear them out.

6. False. Eyes that are "weak" for whatever reason did not become so from overuse, so they cannot be improved by rest.

7. False. Crossed eyes in children should always be considered serious; in fact, the condition requires referral to an ophthalmologist. Some children have apparent but not truly crossed eyes. In such cases, the apparent crossing is due to a broad bridge of the nose in young children. As the nose matures, this apparent crossing lessens and disappears. However, truly crossed eyes should never be ignored, as the condition will not improve with time.

8. False. Incorrectly fitted contact lenses can change the shape of the cornea but do not thereby correct myopia. Intentionally fitting contact lenses incorrectly to change corneal shape can cause permanent harm to the eyes.

9. False. The idea that reading problems are due to poor eye coordination is a misconception, as the results of many controlled studies have indicated.

10. False. Because a cataract is an opacity in the lens of the eye, the cataract cannot grow back when the entire lens is removed (intracapsular extraction). However, the posterior capsule of the lens may

opacify when the lens is not completely removed (extracapsular extraction). This latter technique is nevertheless currently preferred.

11. False. The need for cataract surgery is indicated principally by the degree of functional impairment caused by the cataract, not by any criteria related to its duration.

12. False. All individuals become presbyopic (their eyes lose some of their ability to adjust) with age, regardless of their underlying refractive error.

13. False. The ability of an older person to read without glasses may show only that they have myopia in one eye with reasonably good visual acuity. The nearsightedness could be caused by a cataract. Furthermore, the field of vision could be extremely constricted, as in advanced glaucoma, or one eye could be completely blind.

14. False. Glasses do not affect the health of the eyes. As long as an individual is satisfied with the vision provided by the present glasses, routine visual acuity examinations are generally unnecessary.

15. False. As indicated in some earlier answers, the eye cannot be harmed by the way in which light enters it. The eye merely deals with light, regardless of contrast. Watching television with or without illumination is a matter of comfort rather than harm. An individual who finds the marked contrast of a bright television picture in a dimly lighted room uncomfortable should turn on a light, but neither situation will harm the eyes.

16. False. Eyewash should be used as infrequently as possible. As long as it is functioning properly, the eyes' natural lubrication system is adequate for cleansing them.

17. False. Only the cornea can be transplanted, and the cornea is colorless in all eyes. (The iris gives eyes their color.)

18. False. The conjunctiva prevents a contact lens from passing behind the eye.

19. False. A cataract is an imperfection in the transparency of the normal lens of the eye, not a "growth" or "film" that covers the eye. If the lens becomes opaque enough to significantly impair a person's functional vision, all or most of the lens is surgically removed. Nothing is "peeled" away.

20. False. Headaches are not usually caused by ocular factors.

You will find more detailed and specific rationales for these answers in the various chapters of this text and in the resources suggested at the end of each chapter.

Chapter 1

The Eye Examination

Objectives

As a primary care physician, you should be able to recognize the significant external and internal ocular structures of the normal eye and to perform a basic eye examination.

To achieve these objectives, you should learn

- The essentials of ocular anatomy
- To measure and record visual acuity
- To assess pupillary reflexes
- To evaluate ocular motility
- To use the direct ophthalmoscope for a systematic fundus examination and assessment of the red reflex
- To dilate the pupils as an adjunct to ophthalmoscopy
- To evaluate visual fields by confrontation

Relevance

The proper performance of a basic eye examination is a crucial skill for the primary care physician. Systematic examination of the eye enables the primary care physician to evaluate ocular complaints and provide either definitive treatment or appropriate referral to an ophthalmologist. Furthermore, many eye diseases are "silent," or asymptomatic, while serious ocular damage is occurring. Performing a basic eye examination can reveal such conditions and ensure that patients receive the timely care they need. A basic eye examination may provide early warning signs of any of the following conditions:

- **Blinding eye disease**   Important examples of blinding eye diseases that are potentially treatable if discovered early include cataract, glaucoma, diabetic retinopathy, macular degeneration, and, in young children, amblyopia.
- **Systemic disease**   Potentially life-threatening systemic disorders that may involve the eye include diabetes, hypertension, temporal arteritis, and an embolism from the carotid artery or the heart.
- **Tumor or other disorders of the brain**   These conditions may threaten both vision and life. Important examples include meningioma, aneurysms, and multiple sclerosis.

Basic Information

Figures 1.1 through 1.3 show key external and internal ocular structures. The principal anatomic structures are described below.

Anatomy

- **Eyelids**   The outer structures that protect the eyeball and lubricate the ocular surface. Within each lid is a tarsal plate containing meibomian glands. The lids come together at the medial and lateral canthi. The space between the two open lids is called the *palpebral fissure.*
- **Sclera**   The thick outer coat of the eye, normally white and opaque.
- **Limbus**   The junction between the cornea and the sclera.
- **Iris**   The colored part of the eye that screens out light, primarily via the pigment epithelium, which lines its posterior surface.
- **Pupil**   The circular opening in the center of the iris that adjusts the amount of light entering the eye. Its size is determined by the parasympathetic and sympathetic innervation of the iris.
- **Conjunctiva**   The thin, vascular tissue covering the inner aspect of the eyelids (palpebral conjunctiva) and sclera (bulbar conjunctiva).
- **Cornea**   The transparent front "window" of the eye that serves as the major refractive surface.
- **Extraocular muscles**   The six muscles that move the globe medially (medial rectus), laterally (lateral rectus), upward (superior rectus and inferior oblique), downward (inferior rectus and superior oblique), and torsionally (superior and inferior obliques). These muscles are supplied by three cranial nerves: cranial nerve IV, which innervates the superior oblique; cranial nerve VI, which innervates the lateral rectus; and cranial nerve III, which controls the remainder of the extraocular muscles.
- **Anterior chamber**   The space that lies between the cornea anteriorly and the iris posteriorly. The chamber contains a watery fluid called *aqueous humor.*
- **Lens**   The transparent, biconvex body suspended by the zonules behind the pupil and iris; part of the refracting mechanism of the eye.
- **Ciliary body**   The structure that produces aqueous humor. Contraction of the ciliary muscle changes tension on the zonular fibers that suspend the lens and allows the eye to focus from distant to near objects (accommodation).
- **Posterior chamber**   The small space filled with aqueous humor behind the iris and in front of the vitreous.
- **Vitreous cavity**   The relatively large space (4.5 cc) behind the lens that extends to the retina. The cavity is filled with a transparent jelly-like material called *vitreous humor.*
- **Retina**   The neural tissue lining the vitreous cavity posteriorly. Essentially transparent except for the blood vessels on its inner surface, the retina sends the initial visual signals to the brain via the optic nerve. The retina, macula, choroid, and optic disc are sometimes referred to as the *retinal fundus* or, simply, *fundus.*

- **Macula**   The area of the retina at the posterior pole of the eye responsible for fine, central vision. The oval depression in the center of the macula is called the *fovea*.
- **Choroid**   The vascular, pigmented tissue layer between the sclera and the retina. The choroid provides the blood supply for the outer retinal layers.
- **Optic disc**   The portion of the optic nerve visible within the eye. It is comprised of axons whose cell bodies are located in the ganglion cell layer of the retina.

Optics

The cornea and the lens make up the refractive surfaces of the eye. The cornea provides approximately two thirds of the refractive power of the eye, and the lens approximately one third to form an image on the retina. Reduced visual acuity will result if the axial length of the eye is either too short (ie, *hyperopia*; also called *hypermetropia*) or too long (ie, *myopia*) for the refracting power of the cornea and lens. Visual acuity also is reduced if the refracting power of the cornea and lens is different in one meridian than in another (ie, *astigmatism*). These optical defects can be corrected by the use of either eyeglass lenses or contact lenses. A pinhole placed directly in front of the eye will narrow the effective pupillary aperture and thereby minimize the blurring induced by a refractive error.

The ability of the ciliary muscle to contract and the lens to become more convex is called *accommodation*. With increasing age, the lens of every eye undergoes a progressive hardening, with loss of ability to change its shape. Loss of accommodation is manifested by a decreased ability to focus on near objects (ie, *presbyopia*), while corrected distance visual acuity remains normal. Presbyopia develops progressively with age but becomes clinically manifest in the early to mid 40s, when the ability to accommodate at reading distance (35 to 40 cm) is lost. Presbyopia is corrected by eyeglass lenses, either as reading glasses or as the lower segment of bifocal lenses, the upper segment of which can contain a correction for distance visual acuity if needed. Some myopic patients with presbyopia simply remove their distance glasses to read, because they do not need to accommodate in an uncorrected state.

Visual Acuity

Visual acuity is a measurement of the smallest object a person can identify at a given distance from the eye. The following are common abbreviations used to discuss visual acuity:

- VA   visual acuity
- OD   (*oculus dexter*) right eye
- OS   (*oculus sinister*) left eye
- OU   (*oculus uterque*) both eyes

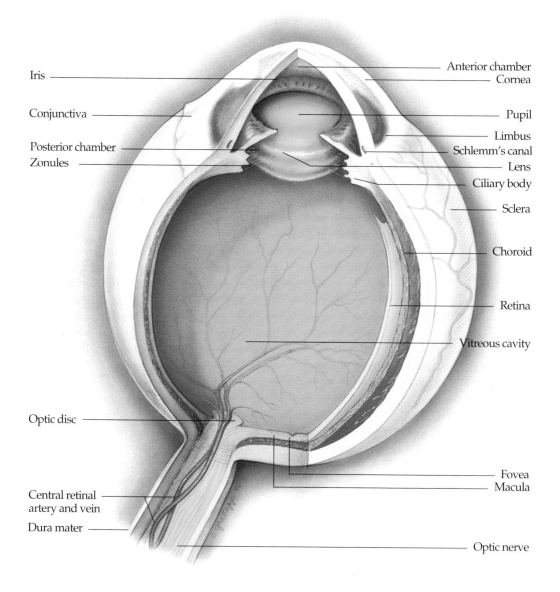

Iris

Conjunctiva

Posterior chamber
Zonules

Anterior chamber
Cornea

Pupil

Limbus
Schlemm's canal
Lens
Ciliary body

Sclera

Choroid

Retina

Vitreous cavity

Optic disc

Central retinal
artery and vein
Dura mater

Fovea
Macula

Optic nerve

Figure 1.1 Cross-section of the eye. (Courtesy Christine Gralapp.)

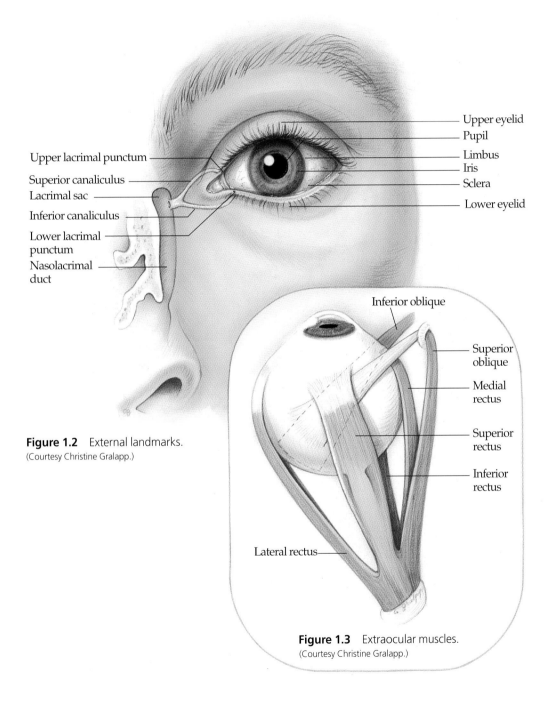

Upper eyelid
Pupil
Limbus
Iris
Sclera
Lower eyelid

Upper lacrimal punctum
Superior canaliculus
Lacrimal sac
Inferior canaliculus
Lower lacrimal punctum
Nasolacrimal duct

Figure 1.2   External landmarks.
(Courtesy Christine Gralapp.)

Inferior oblique

Superior oblique
Medial rectus
Superior rectus
Inferior rectus

Lateral rectus

Figure 1.3   Extraocular muscles.
(Courtesy Christine Gralapp.)

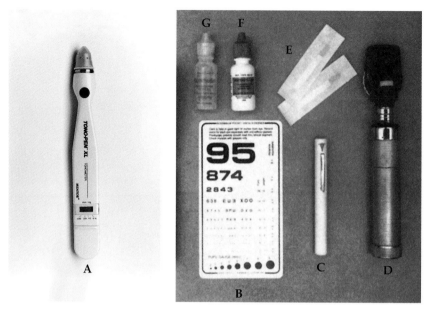

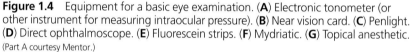

Figure 1.4 Equipment for a basic eye examination. (**A**) Electronic tonometer (or other instrument for measuring intraocular pressure). (**B**) Near vision card. (**C**) Penlight. (**D**) Direct ophthalmoscope. (**E**) Fluorescein strips. (**F**) Mydriatic. (**G**) Topical anesthetic. (Part A courtesy Mentor.)

When to Examine

All patients should have an eye examination as part of a general physical examination by the primary care physician. Visual acuity, pupillary reactions, extraocular movements, and direct ophthalmoscopy through undilated pupils constitute a minimal examination. Pupillary dilation for ophthalmoscopy is required in cases of unexplained visual loss or when fundus pathology is suspected (eg, diabetes mellitus).

Distance visual acuity measurement should be performed in all children as soon as possible after age 3 because of the importance of detecting amblyopia early. The tumbling E chart (see Chapter 6) is used in place of the standard Snellen eye chart.

Depending on what the examination reveals and on the patient's history, additional tests may be indicated (listed below). Details on how to perform both basic and adjunctive ocular tests appear in the following section, "How to Examine."

Additional Tests

- **Tonometry** Should be performed as clinically indicated whenever the diagnosis of glaucoma is suspected.
- **Anterior chamber depth assessment** Indicated when narrow-angle glaucoma is suspected and prior to pupillary dilation.
- **Confrontation field testing** May be suggested by the patient's history or symptoms to confirm a suspected field defect.

- **Color vision testing**   May be part of an eye examination when requested by the patient or by another agency and in patients with retinal or optic nerve disorders.
- **Fluorescein staining**   Is necessary when a corneal epithelial defect or abnormality is suspected.
- **Eversion of the upper lid**   Is necessary when the presence of a foreign body is suspected.

How to Examine

Equipment for an eye examination consists of a few items that can be transported, if necessary, with other medical instruments (Figure 1.4). The slit-lamp biomicroscope is a stationary office instrument that augments the inspection of the anterior segment of the eye by providing an illuminated, magnified view. Standard equipment in an ophthalmologist's office, the slit lamp is also available in many emergency facilities.

Distance Visual Acuity Testing

Distance visual acuity is usually recorded as a ratio or fraction comparing patient performance with an agreed-upon standard. In this notation, the first number represents the distance between the patient and the eye chart (usually the Snellen eye chart, Figure 1.5); the second number represents the distance at which the letters can be read by a person with normal acuity. Visual acuity of 20/80 thus indicates that the patient can recognize at 20 feet a symbol that can be recognized by a person with normal acuity at 80 feet.

Visual acuity of 20/20 represents normal visual acuity. Many "normal" individuals actually see better than 20/20—for example, 20/15 or even 20/12. If this is the case, you should record it as such. Alternative notations are the decimal notation (eg, 20/20 = 1.0; 20/40 = 0.5; 20/200 = 0.1) and the metric notation (eg, 20/20 = 6/6, 20/100 = 6/30).

Visual acuity is tested most often at a distance of 20 feet, or 6 meters. Greater distances are cumbersome and impractical; at shorter distances, variations in the test distance assume greater proportional significance. For practical purposes, a distance of 20 feet may be equated with optical infinity.

To test distance visual acuity with the conventional Snellen eye chart, follow these steps:

1. Place the patient at the designated distance, usually 20 feet (6 meters), from a well-illuminated Snellen chart (see Figure 1.5). If glasses are normally worn for distance vision, the patient should wear them.
2. By convention, the right eye is tested and recorded first. Completely occlude the left eye using an opaque occluder or the palm of your hand; alternatively, have the patient cover the eye.

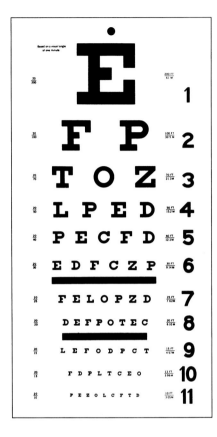

Figure 1.5   Snellen eye chart.

3. Ask the patient to read the smallest line in which he can distinguish more than one half of the letters. (If the E chart is being used, have the patient designate the direction in which the strokes of the E point.)
4. Record the acuity measurement as a notation (eg, 20/20) in which the first number represents the distance at which the test is performed and the second number represents the numeric designation for the line read.
5. Repeat the procedure for the other eye.
6. If visual acuity is 20/40 or less in one or both eyes, repeat the test with the subject viewing the test chart through a pinhole occluder and record these results. The pinhole occluder may be used over the subject's glasses.

If a patient cannot see the largest Snellen letters, proceed as follows:

1. Reduce the distance between the patient and the chart. Record the new distance as the numerator of the acuity designation (eg, 5/70).
2. If the patient is unable to see the largest Snellen letter at 3 feet, hold up one hand, extend two or more fingers, and ask the patient to count the number of fingers. Record the distance at which counting fingers is done accurately (eg, CF 1 ft).
3. If the patient cannot count fingers, determine whether or not he can detect the movement of your hand. Record a positive response as hand motion (eg, HM 2 ft).

4. If the patient cannot detect hand motion, use a penlight to determine whether he can detect the presence or direction of light. Record the patient's response as LP (light perception), LP with projection (light perception with direction), or NLP (no light perception).

Visual Impairment vs Visual Disability

The term *visual acuity impairment* (or simply *visual impairment*) is used to describe a condition of the eyes. *Visual disability* describes a condition of the individual. The disabling effect of an impairment depends in part on the individual's ability to adapt and to compensate. Two individuals with the same visual impairment measured on a Snellen eye chart may show very different levels of functional disability. Table 1.1 summarizes the differences between visual impairment and visual disability.

Table 1.1   Visual Impairment vs Visual Disability

Visual Impairment	Visual Disability	Comment
20/12 to 20/25	Normal vision	Healthy young adults average better than 20/20 acuity.
20/30 to 20/70	Near-normal vision	Usually causes no serious problems, but vision should be explored for potential improvement or possible early disease. Most states will issue a driver's license to individuals with this level of vision in at least one eye.
20/80 to 20/160	Moderate low vision	Strong reading glasses or vision magnifiers usually provide adequate reading ability; this level is usually insufficient for a driver's license.
20/200 to 20/400 or CF 10 ft	Severe low vision; legal blindness by US definition	Gross orientation and mobility generally adequate, but difficulty with traffic signs, bus numbers, etc. Reading requires high-power magnifiers; reading speed reduced.
CF 8 ft to 4 ft	Profound low vision	Increasing problems with visual orientation and mobility. Long cane useful to explore environment. Highly motivated and persistent individuals can read with extreme magnification. Others rely on nonvisual communication: braille, "talking books," radio, etc.
Less than CF 4 ft	Near-total blindness	Vision unreliable, except under ideal circumstances; must rely on nonvisual aids.
NLP	Total blindness	No light perception; must rely entirely on other senses.

Near Visual Acuity Testing

Near visual acuity testing may be performed if the patient has a complaint about near vision. Otherwise, testing "at near" is performed only if distance testing is difficult or impossible—at the patient's bedside, for instance. In such situations, testing with a near card may be the only feasible way to determine visual acuity.

If the patient normally wears glasses for reading, he should wear them during testing. This holds true for the presbyopic patient in particular. The patient holds the test card—for example, a Rosenbaum pocket vision screener (Figure 1.6)—at the distance specified on the card. This distance is usually 14 inches or 35 centimeters. While the examiner occludes one of the patient's eyes, the patient reads the smallest characters legible on the card. The test is then repeated for the other eye.

Letter size designations and test distances vary. To avoid ambiguity, both should be recorded (eg, J5 at 14 in, 6 point at 40 cm). Some near cards carry distance-equivalent values. These are valid only if the test is done at the recommended distance. If a standard near vision card is not available, any printed matter such as a telephone book or a newspaper may be substituted. Both the approximate type size read and the distance at which the material was held are recorded.

Visual Acuity Estimation in an Uncooperative Patient

Occasionally, you will encounter a patient who is unwilling or unable to cooperate with standard visual acuity testing or who may be suspected of faking blindness. Because the typical visual acuity test will not work for such a patient, you will need to be alert to other signs. Withdrawal or a change in facial expression in response to light or sudden movement indicates the presence of vision. A brisk pupillary response to light also suggests the presence of vision. The exception to this is the patient with cortical blindness, which is due to bilateral widespread destruction of the visual cortex. If there is any doubt, referral to an ophthalmologist is recommended.

Chapter 6 discusses visual testing of infants and toddlers.

External Inspection

With adequate room light, the examiner can inspect the lids, surrounding tissues, and palpebral fissure. Palpation of the orbital rim and lids may be indicated, depending on the history and symptoms. Inspection of the conjunctiva and sclera is facilitated by using a penlight and having the patient look up while the examiner retracts the lower lid or look down while the examiner raises the upper lid. The penlight also aids in the inspection of both the cornea and the iris.

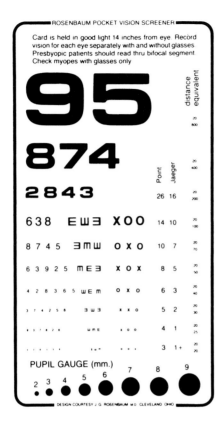

ROSENBAUM POCKET VISION SCREENER

Figure 1.6   Rosenbaum pocket vision screener.

Pupillary Reaction Testing

Inspection of the pupils should be part of the physical examination. The patient's direct and consensual pupillary reactions to light are evaluated in a room with reduced illumination and with the patient looking at a distant object.

To test the direct pupillary reaction to light, first direct the penlight at the patient's right eye and see if it constricts (a normal reaction). Repeat for the left pupil. To test the consensual pupillary reaction to light, direct the penlight at the right eye and watch the left pupil to see if it constricts along with the right pupil (a normal consensual response). Repeat for the left pupil, watching the right pupil for the response. Occasionally, this examination may reveal indications of neurologic disease. (See Chapter 7 for a description of the swinging-flashlight test for the detection of an afferent defect in the anterior visual pathway.) Pupillary inspection may reveal active or prior ocular disease with alterations in pupillary shape or size that are the result of local intraocular processes (eg, damage to the pupillary sphincter or adhesion of the iris to the lens).

Ocular Motility Testing

The patient is asked to follow an object in six directions, the cardinal fields of gaze:

1. Right and up   4. Left and up
2. Right   5. Left
3. Right and down   6. Left and down

This enables the examiner to systematically test each muscle in its primary field of action (Table 1.2). Thus, a possible isolated weakness or paralysis of muscle can best be detected. (See Chapter 6 for a description of the cover test for the detection of strabismus, a misalignment of the two eyes.)

Ophthalmoscopy

When examining the patient's right eye, hold the direct ophthalmoscope in the right hand and use your right eye to view the patient's eye. Use your left hand and left eye to examine the patient's left eye. The patient's eyeglasses are removed, and, barring large astigmatic refractive errors, most examiners prefer to remove their own glasses as well. Contact lenses worn by either patient or examiner may be left in place.

Pupillary Dilation

Pharmacologic dilation of the patient's pupils greatly facilitates ophthalmoscopy. Recommended agents include tropicamide 1% and phenylephrine hydrochloride 2.5% (see Chapter 9). Dilation of the pupil should not be done under the following conditions:

1. If assessment of anterior chamber depth suggests a shallow chamber and a narrow angle, do not dilate because an attack of angle-closure glaucoma might be precipitated.
2. If a patient is undergoing neurologic observation and pupillary signs are being watched (eg, a head-injured patient), do not dilate until the neurologist or neurosurgeon determines it is safe to do so.

Table 1.2   Cardinal Fields of Gaze

Right and Up	**Left and Up**
Right superior rectus	Left superior rectus
Left inferior oblique	Right inferior oblique
Right	**Left**
Right lateral rectus	Left lateral rectus
Left medial rectus	Right medical rectus
Right and Down	**Left and Down**
Right inferior rectus	Left inferior rectus
Left superior oblique	Right superior oblique

3. If a patient has had a cataract extraction with implantation of an iris-supported intraocular lens, do not dilate because the lens implant could dislocate. The iris-supported intraocular lens was a popular implant at one time but is no longer available, although many individuals still retain these implants in their eyes. The pupil in such a patient is usually square-shaped.

See Chapter 9 for instructions on applying topical agents.

Method of Direct Ophthalmoscopy

To perform direct ophthalmoscopy, follow these steps:

1. Have the patient comfortably seated. Instruct the patient to look at a point on the wall straight ahead, trying not to move the eyes.
2. Set the focusing wheel at about +8. Set the aperture wheel to select the large, round, white light.
3. Begin to look at the right eye about 1 foot from the patient. Use your right eye with the ophthalmoscope in your right hand. When you look straight down the patient's line of sight at the pupil, you will see the red reflex (see below).
4. Place your free hand on the patient's forehead or shoulder to aid your proprioception and to keep yourself steady.
5. Slowly come close to the patient at an angle of about 15° temporal to the patient's line of sight. Try to keep the pupil in view. Turn the focusing wheel to bring the patient's retina into focus.
6. When a retinal vessel comes into view, follow it as it widens to the optic disc, which lies nasal to the center of the retina.
7. Examine the optic disc, retinal blood vessels, retinal background, and macula in that order (see below).
8. Repeat for the left eye.

Red Reflex

Light reflected off the fundus of the patient produces a red reflex when viewed through the ophthalmoscope at a distance of 1 foot. A normal red reflex (Slide 1) is evenly colored and is not interrupted by shadows. Opacities in the media appear as black silhouettes and can be best appreciated when the pupil has been dilated (see Slide 17 in Chapter 3).

Optic Disc

In most cases, when viewed through the ophthalmoscope, the normal optic disc (Slide 2) is slightly oval in the vertical meridian and has a pink color. A central depression in the surface of the disc is called the *physiologic cup*. The optic disc can be thought of as the yardstick of the ocular fundus. Lesions seen with the ophthalmoscope are measured in disc diameters (1 disc diameter equals approximately 1.5 mm).

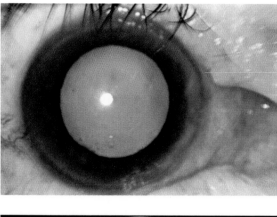

Slide 1   Red reflex. Reddish light reflected from the fundus can be visible even at a distance of 1 or 2 feet when the direction of illumination and the direction of observation approach each other—a condition that can be achieved with the ophthalmoscope.

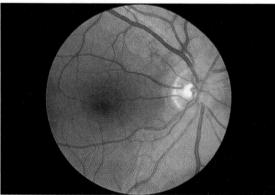

Slide 2   Normal posterior pole. A normal optic disc is shown, with a small central physiologic cup and healthy neural rim. Major branches of the central retinal artery emanate from the disc, whereas the major branches of the central retinal vein collect at the disc. Temporal to the disc is the macula, which appears darker; no blood vessels are present in the center.

A great deal of normal variation exists in the appearance of the optic disc. The size of the physiologic cup varies among individuals. (See Chapter 3 for a discussion of glaucomatous cupping.) The pigmented coats of the eye—the retinal pigment epithelium and the choroid—frequently fail to reach the margin of the optic disc, producing a hypopigmented crescent (Slide 3, left). Such crescents are especially common in myopic eyes on the temporal side of the optic disc. Conversely, an excess of pigment may be seen in some eyes, producing a heavily pigmented margin along the optic disc (see Slide 3, right). The retinal nerve fibers (ie, ganglion cell axons) ordinarily are nonmyelinated at the optic disc and in the retina, but occasionally myelination may extend onto the surface of the optic disc and retina, producing a dense, white superficial opacification with feathery edges (Slide 4).

Retinal Circulation

The retinal circulation is composed of arteries and veins, visible with the ophthalmoscope (compare Figure 1.7 with Slide 2). The central retinal artery branches at or on the optic disc into divisions that supply the four quadrants of the inner retinal layers; these divisions lie superficially in the

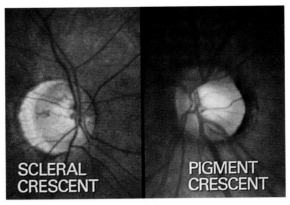

Slide 3   Scleral crescent and pigmented crescent. This figure shows normal variants of the optic disc. On the left, retinal and choroidal pigmentation does not reach the disc margin, leaving an exposed white scleral crescent. On the right, pigment accumulation is seen at the disc margin.

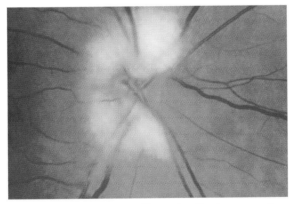

Slide 4   Myelinated nerve fibers. Usually, the axons of the retinal ganglion cells acquire myelin sheaths only behind the optic disc. Occasionally, as a variant, myelin is deposited along axons at the border of the disc or even away from the disc, elsewhere in the retina. These white, feathery patterns may be mistaken for papilledema.

nerve fiber layer. A similarly arranged system of retinal veins collects at the optic disc, where spontaneous pulsation (with collapse during systole) may be observed in 80% of normal eyes. The ratio of normal vein-to-artery diameter is 3:2. Arteries are usually lighter in color than veins and typically have a more prominent light reflex from their surfaces than do veins. The examiner should follow arteries from the disc and veins back to the disc in each quadrant, noting in particular the arteriovenous (A/V) crossing patterns.

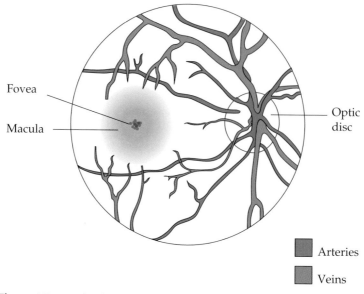

Arteries

Veins

Figure 1.7 Fundus diagram.

Retinal Background

The normal retinal background is a uniform red-orange color due primarily to the pigmentation of the retinal pigment epithelium. The blood and pigment of the choroid also contribute to the appearance of the retinal background. For example, in heavily pigmented eyes, the fundus may have a darker color due to increased choroidal pigment content.

Macula

The normal macula (see Figure 1.7 and Slide 2), located directly temporal and slightly inferior to the optic disc, usually appears darker than the surrounding retina because the specialized retinal pigment epithelial cells of the macula are taller and more heavily pigmented. In some eyes, the macula may appear slightly yellow due to the xanthophyll pigment in the retina. The central depression of the fovea may act as a concave mirror during ophthalmoscopy and produce a light reflection known as the *foveal reflex*.

Intraocular Pressure Measurement

Intraocular pressure (IOP) is determined largely by the outflow of aqueous humor from the eye. The greater the resistance to outflow, the higher the intraocular pressure. Alterations in the actual production of aqueous humor also have an effect on the intraocular pressure.

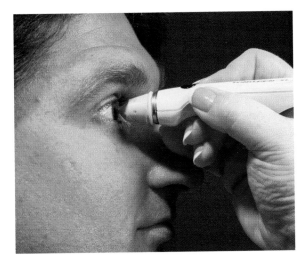

Figure 1.8 Electronic tonometry. Electronic tonometry can be performed with the patient in any position. (Courtesy Mentor.)

Intraocular pressure varies among individuals. An IOP of 15 millimeters of mercury (mm Hg) represents the mean in a "normal" population. However, an IOP in the range from 10 to 21 mm Hg falls within 2 standard deviations of the mean.

Measurement of IOP is an essential part of a glaucoma screening examination, along with ophthalmoscopic assessment of the optic cup. IOP determination is especially helpful for diagnosing patients in the early stages of chronic open-angle glaucoma, when pressure is elevated but pathologic cupping has not yet developed. IOP determination is also useful when the diagnosis of acute angle-closure glaucoma is being considered.

In the past, the Schiøtz (indentation) tonometer has been used by primary care physicians to measure intraocular pressure. Schiøtz tonometry is an inexpensive and simple method of measuring intraocular pressure and, if available, can be used to measure the intraocular pressure in a patient with suspected angle-closure glaucoma. With the patient in a supine position, the Schiøtz device with a given weight is placed on the patient's anesthetized cornea and indents the cornea in an amount related to the IOP. A printed conversion table that accompanies the tonometer is used to determine the IOP in millimeters of mercury.

Currently, handheld electronic tonometers are available in some hospital emergency departments to measure intraocular pressure (Figure 1.8). One such device is brand-named Tono-Pen. An electronic tonometer is a solid-state strain gauge that converts the IOP to an electrical signal. This battery-operated device weighs just a few ounces and can be used with the patient in any position, as opposed to other devices that require the patient to be either seated or supine. The intraocular pressure results are obtained rapidly with the electronic tonometer and correlate highly with those obtained by the Goldmann applanation tonometer. Electronic tonometers are expensive and require daily calibration.

To perform electronic tonometry, the practitioner instills topical anesthetic in the patient's eyes and, starting with the patient's right eye, separates the lids and applies the calibrated tonometer to the patient's cornea. The pressure reading and reliability rating displayed on the device are noted in the patient's record.

Topical anesthetics applied for tonometry have little effect on the margins of the eyelids. If the tonometer touches the lids, the patient will feel it and squeeze the lids together, impeding IOP measurement. This can be avoided by holding the patient's lids wide apart with the free hand while applying the tonometer tip with the other hand. Take care not to apply digital pressure to the eyeball while holding the lids apart, as it may produce a falsely high pressure reading. Tonometry should never be attempted in a patient suspected of having a ruptured globe; doing so could result in further damage to the eye.

Anterior Chamber Depth Assessment

When the anterior chamber is shallow, the iris becomes convex as it is bowed forward over the lens. Under these conditions, the nasal iris is seen in shadow when a light is directed from the opposite side (Figure 1.9). As the shallowness of the anterior chamber increases, so do the convexity of the iris and the shaded view of the nasal iris. A shallow anterior chamber may indicate narrow-angle glaucoma (also called *angle-closure glaucoma*) or a narrow angle that could close with pupillary dilation.

To assess anterior chamber depth, follow these steps:

1. Shine a light from the temporal side of the head across the front of the eye parallel to the plane of the iris.
2. Look at the nasal aspect of the iris. If two thirds or more of the nasal iris is in shadow, the chamber is probably shallow and the angle narrow.

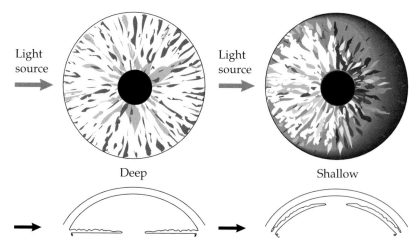

Figure 1.9   Estimation of anterior chamber depth.

3. If you are unsure of the extent of shadow, direct the light more from the front of the eye, which will eliminate shadows entirely, and then return the light to the temporal side of the head.
4. Repeat the test for the other eye.

Confrontation Field Testing

The examiner takes a position in front of the patient. The patient is asked to cover the left eye with the palm of the left hand; the examiner closes the right eye. Thus, the field of the examiner's left eye is used as a reference in assessing the field of the patient's right eye. The patient is asked to fixate on the examiner's left eye and then count the fingers of the examiner in each of the four quadrants of the visual field. Wiggling the fingers as a visual stimulus is not desirable. After the patient's right eye is tested, the procedure is repeated for the left eye, with the patient covering the right eye with the palm of the right hand, and the examiner closing the left eye.

Amsler Grid Testing

Amsler grid testing is a method of evaluating the functioning of the macula. (See Figure 3.4 and Chapter 3 for details.)

Color Vision Testing

The normal retina contains three color-sensitive pigments: red-sensitive, green-sensitive, and blue-sensitive. A developmental deficiency in either the concentration or the function of one or more of these pigments causes various combinations and degrees of congenital color vision defects. Most such defects occur in males through an X-linked inheritance pattern. Color vision abnormalities also may be acquired in individuals with retinal or optic nerve disorders.

Color vision testing is performed with the use of pseudoisochromatic plates (eg, Ishihara plates), which present numbers or figures against a background of colored dots. The person with abnormal color discrimination will be confused by the pseudoisochromatic plates, which force a choice based on hue discrimination alone while concealing other clues such as brightness, saturation, and contours.

The patient should wear glasses during color vision testing if they are normally worn for near vision. The color plates are presented consecutively under good illumination, preferably natural light. Results are recorded according to the detailed instructions provided with the plates. Usually, a fraction is specified, with the numerator equivalent to the number of correct responses and the denominator the total plates presented. The type of color defect can be determined by recording the specific errors and using the instructions provided with the plates.

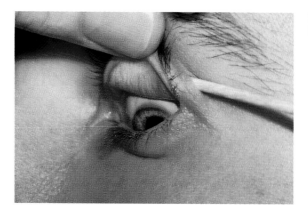

Figure 1.10
Upper lid eversion.

Upper Lid Eversion

Upper lid eversion is sometimes required to search for conjunctival foreign bodies or other conjunctival signs. Topical anesthetic facilitates this procedure. The patient is asked to look down and the examiner grasps the eyelashes of the upper lid between the thumb and the index finger. A cotton-tipped applicator is used to press gently downward over the superior aspect of the tarsal plate as the lid margin is pulled upward by the lashes (Figure 1.10). Pressure is maintained on the everted upper lid while the patient is encouraged to keep looking down. The examiner should have a penlight within reach to inspect the exposed conjunctival surface of the upper lid for a foreign body or other abnormality. A cotton-tipped applicator soaked in topical anesthetic can be used to remove a foreign body. To return the lid to its normal position, the examiner releases the lid margin and the patient is instructed to look up.

Fluorescein Staining of Cornea

Corneal staining with fluorescein (a yellow-green dye) is useful in diagnosing defects of the corneal epithelium. Fluorescein is applied in the form of a sterile filter-paper strip, which is moistened with a drop of sterile water, saline, or topical anesthetic and then touched to the palpebral conjunctiva. A few blinks spread the fluorescein over the cornea. Areas of bright-green staining denote absent or diseased epithelium (Slide 5). Viewing the eye under cobalt-blue light enhances the visibility of the fluorescence (Slide 6).

Two precautions to keep in mind when using fluorescein are

1. Use fluorescein-impregnated strips instead of stock solutions of fluorescein because such solutions are susceptible to contamination with *Pseudomonas* species.
2. Have the patient remove soft contact lenses prior to application to avoid discoloration of the lenses.

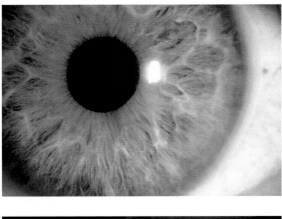

Slide 5 Fluorescein stain. A corneal abrasion is delineated by fluorescein stain, which marks any area denuded of epithelium. Irregularity of the corneal surface is indicated by the distorted light reflection.

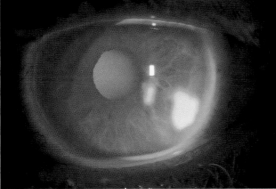

Slide 6 Fluorescein stain highlighted. The addition of cobalt-blue light dramatically defines the corneal epithelial defect.

Summary of Steps in Eye Examination

1. Measure the visual acuity for each eye.
2. Perform a confrontation field test for each eye.
3. Inspect the lids and the surrounding tissues.
4. Inspect the conjunctiva and sclera.
5. Test the extraocular movements.
6. Test the pupils for direct and consensual responses.
7. Inspect the cornea and iris.
8. Assess the anterior chamber for depth and clarity.
9. Assess the lens for clarity through direct ophthalmoscopy.
10. Use the ophthalmoscope to study the fundus, including the disc, vessels, and macula.
11. Perform tonometry when indicated.

Management or
Referral

Reduced Visual Acuity

The guidelines below apply for patients in whom reduced visual acuity is found, unless the patient has been seen by an ophthalmologist and the condition has been confirmed as stable.

- **VA less than 20/20**   Any patient with visual acuity less than 20/20 in one or both eyes should be referred to an ophthalmologist if visual symptoms are present. Reduced visual acuity is the best single criterion by which to differentiate potentially blinding conditions from less serious ocular disorders.
- **VA less than 20/40**   Any patient with visual acuity less than 20/40 in both eyes is an equally important candidate for referral, even in the absence of complaints. Although many such patients suffer only from uncorrected refractive errors, undetected painless but progressive loss of vision does occur in many disorders of the eyes and visual system.
- **Asymmetry**   Any patient with a difference in visual acuity between the eyes of 2 lines or more on the Snellen chart should be referred promptly, even if visual acuity in one or both eyes is better than 20/40. Generally, visual function is nearly identical between the eyes; thus, in the absence of known causes of reduced vision, asymmetry of visual acuity may be a sign of occult disease.
- **Presbyopia**   Presbyopia is manifested by reduced near vision with no change in distance visual acuity. Middle-aged or elderly patients complaining of this combination will benefit from a referral for the prescription of corrective lenses.

Abnormal Fundus
Appearance

Only after performing numerous fundus examinations will the practitioner be able to recognize the great range of normal ophthalmoscopic appearances. When an abnormality is suspected, further studies or consultation may be required because fundus abnormalities can indicate significant ocular or systemic diseases. Ophthalmologic consultation should be sought for fundus changes accompanied by acute or chronic visual complaints.

Photographs of the fundus are taken with a special camera that provides a greater field of view than is possible with the direct ophthalmoscope. Many fundus abnormalities have three-dimensional qualities, such as elevation or depression, but the examiner is limited to a monocular, two-dimensional view with the direct ophthalmoscope. It is necessary to learn to think in three dimensions in order to grasp the pathophysiology.

Shallow Anterior Chamber Depth/Elevated Intraocular Pressure

A patient suspected of having shallow anterior chamber depth (at risk for angle-closure glaucoma) or documented intraocular pressure of 22 mm Hg or greater should be referred to an ophthalmologist for further evaluation.

Points to Remember

1. To prevent patients from reading the visual acuity chart with both eyes, either intentionally or unintentionally, the examiner must ensure that one eye is completely occluded.
2. A well-lighted hallway often provides an acceptable location for distance visual acuity testing with a standard Snellen chart.
3. To avoid measurement error when performing tonometry, the examiner must keep the lids apart by holding them firmly against the bony margins of the orbit, rather than by pressing them against the globe.

Sample Problems

1. A 14-year-old boy is seen for a physical examination at school. He admits to difficulty in reading the blackboard but not in reading textbooks. He does not wear glasses. You record VA as OD 20/100, pinhole 20/25; and OS 20/100, pinhole 20/25. What is your diagnosis? Would you manage or refer this patient?

   Answer: The combination of decreased distance vision with preserved near vision is typical of myopia, which often becomes symptomatic during adolescence. Presumptive evidence of refractive error is provided by the marked improvement in visual acuity that occurs with the use of the pinhole. Note that visual acuity with pinhole frequently does not reach 20/20. The patient should be referred to an ophthalmologist as a regular rather than an urgent consultation.

2. A 78-year-old woman is seen for an annual physical examination and complains of mild difficulty in reading and seeing street signs. You record OD 20/70, no improvement with pinhole; and OS 20/50, no improvement with pinhole. Upon direct ophthalmoscopy, you note a dullness of the red reflex and you have difficulty seeing fundus details in both eyes. What is your diagnosis? Would you manage or refer this patient?

   Answer: Cataract is a common cause of painless progressive loss of vision in older individuals. Her complaints about her visual ability are an indication for referral to an ophthalmologist for evaluation for possible cataract surgery.

3. A 40-year-old man is seen for an annual executive physical. He has no complaints and does not wear glasses. You record VA as OD 20/15; and OS 20/100, no improvement with pinhole. During examination, the patient revealed that he has been aware since childhood that his left eye was a so-called lazy eye—in other words, that he suffered from amblyopia. Would you refer this patient?

Answer: Referral is not indicated since the cause of decreased vision is established and progressive loss is not occurring. Note that this healthy individual has better than 20/20 acuity in his right eye.

4. A 50-year-old man visits your office because he noted decreased visual acuity in the right eye the preceding day while accidentally occluding his left eye. When his present glasses were prescribed 2 years ago, his vision was equal in both eyes. You record VA as OD 20/50, no improvement with pinhole; and OS 20/20. Upon ophthalmoscopy, no abnormalities are detected. What, if any, is your diagnosis? Would you manage or refer this patient?

Answer: The patient has an unexplained loss of vision of unknown duration in one eye. An unexplained decrease in vision in one or both eyes requires referral to an ophthalmologist, because it may indicate occult disease of the eyes or central nervous system that is not detectable by examination methods available to the primary care physician. In this case, the patient's decreased vision was due to a macular disturbance detectable only by more precise methods of examination (eg, special lenses and fluorescein angiography).

5. A 55-year-old man, wearing goggles, was sawing wood in his garage shop. He removed the goggles to clean up and, while sweeping up small wood chips, had the sudden onset of a foreign-body sensation in his right eye. The irritation was not relieved with artificial tears, and it intensified with every blink. His wife rushed him to their family doctor for emergency treatment. The physician was able to examine him after placing a topical anesthetic in the right eye. Visual acuity in the right eye was 20/80. Fluorescein staining revealed multiple vertical linear abrasions of the cornea.

A. Explain the clinical findings.

Answer: By history, this man has been exposed to small particles that could abrade his eye. The vertical linear abrasions in conjunction with the feeling of irritation with each blink imply the presence of a foreign body under the upper lid.

B. What further examination is required, and how is it performed?

Answer: Eversion of the upper lid (see page 20) will expose the foreign body, which can then be removed using a cotton-tipped applicator stick.

Annotated Resources

Gittinger JW Jr: *Ophthalmology: A Clinical Introduction*. Boston: Little, Brown & Co; 1984. Chapter 1, "Ocular History and Examination," covers the eye examination in this excellent introductory text for medical students.

Keltner JL, Wand M, Van Newkirk MR: *Techniques for the Basic Ocular Examination*. San Francisco: American Academy of Ophthalmology; 1989. This videotape covers visual acuity testing, ocular motility testing, confrontation field testing, glaucoma screening, and funduscopic examination.

Newell FW: *Ophthalmology: Principles and Concepts*. 8th ed. St Louis: CV Mosby Co; 1996. This comprehensive text covers in detail anatomy (Chapter 1), physiology (Chapter 2), symptoms of eye disease (Chapter 4), and examination techniques (Chapters 5 and 6).

Pavan-Langston D: *Manual of Ocular Diagnosis and Therapy*. 4th ed. Boston: Little, Brown & Co; 1995. Chapter 1, "Ocular Examination Techniques and Diagnostic Tests," of this spiral-bound manual covers the full gamut of techniques, including those that would be used only by an ophthalmologist.

Trobe JD: *The Physician's Guide to Eye Care*. San Francisco: American Academy of Ophthalmology; 1993. This brief but comprehensive and well-illustrated resource covers the principal clinical ophthalmic problems that nonophthalmologist physicians are likely to encounter, organized for practical use by practitioners. Chapter 1 presents techniques for performing a screening examination, and Chapter 2 outlines rationale, frequency, and components of the routine examination for asymptomatic patients.

Vaughan DG, Asbury T, Riordan-Eva P: *General Ophthalmology*. 14th ed. Norwalk, CT: Appleton & Lange; 1995. This is a useful and popular textbook for medical students, ophthalmology residents, and other physicians. Chapter 1, "Anatomy & Embryology of the Eye," contains good anatomic illustrations; Chapter 2, "Ophthalmologic Examination," contains information on ophthalmic instruments and examination techniques.

Wilson FM II, ed: *Practical Ophthalmology: A Manual for Beginning Ophthalmology Residents*. San Francisco: American Academy of Ophthalmology; 1996. Intended for beginning ophthalmology residents, this comprehensive book presents numerous step-by-step protocols for a wide range of basic ophthalmologic examinations, which medical students and residents may find useful.

Chapter 2

Acute Visual Loss

Objectives

As a primary care physician, you should be able to evaluate a patient complaining of a sudden decrease in visual acuity or visual field, to construct a differential diagnosis, and to recognize situations requiring urgent action.

To achieve these objectives, you should learn

- Which questions to ask the patient
- To utilize appropriate examination techniques, with special attention to pupillary responses, visual field testing, and ophthalmoscopy
- Which conditions are most likely to cause acute visual loss

Relevance

For most people, sudden blindness is a paradigm of disaster. The primary care physician needs to recognize the conditions responsible for acute visual loss in order to make urgent referrals to an ophthalmologist and to actually initiate therapy, when appropriate. The ultimate visual outcome may well depend on early, accurate diagnosis and timely treatment.

Basic Information

Important patient history questions to ask in the event of sudden visual loss include

- Is the visual loss transient or persistent?
- Is the visual loss monocular or binocular?
- What was the tempo? Did the visual loss occur abruptly, or did it develop over hours, days, or weeks?
- What are the patient's age and medical condition?
- Did the patient have documented normal vision in the past?

How to Examine

Visual Acuity Testing

The first thing to be determined in evaluating acute visual loss is the visual acuity, with best available correction, in each eye. For detailed information on visual acuity testing, see Chapter 1.

Confrontation Field Testing

Normal acuity does not assure that significant vision has not been lost, because the entire visual field, including peripheral vision, must be considered. For instance, a patient who has lost all of the peripheral vision on one side in both eyes—a homonymous hemianopia—generally has normal visual acuity. For instruction on assessing the visual field through confrontation field testing, see Chapter 1.

Pupillary Reactions

The reaction of the pupils to light is useful in the evaluation of visual loss, especially when that reaction is asymmetric. In the swinging-flashlight test, a bright light is moved from one eye to the other and the pupillary reactions are observed. When there is a lesion in the retina or the optic nerve of one eye, the brain-stem centers controlling pupillary size perceive the light as being brighter in the normal eye. Thus, when the light beam is moved from the normal eye to the abnormal eye, the pupil of the abnormal eye may continue to dilate. This positive swinging-flashlight test indicates a relative afferent pupillary defect, also known as a Marcus Gunn pupil. The presence or absence of a relative afferent pupillary defect is often an important piece of information in the evaluation of monocular visual loss. For more information on pupillary reactions and the swinging-flashlight test, see Chapter 7.

Ophthalmoscopy

Ophthalmoscopy is probably the most important examination technique in the evaluation of visual loss because it allows direct inspection of the fundus and an assessment of the clarity of the refractive media. For information on the technique of direct ophthalmoscopy, see Chapter 1.

Penlight Examination

Simple penlight examination usually will detect corneal disease responsible for acute visual loss.

Tonometry

Tonometry to measure intraocular pressure may help confirm the presence of angle-closure glaucoma.

How to Interpret the Findings

Media Opacities

Any significant irregularity or opacity of the clear refractive media of the eye (cornea, anterior chamber, lens, vitreous) will cause blurred vision or a reduction of visual acuity. These opacities do not cause relative afferent pupillary defects, although pupillary reflexes may be altered (eg, miosis in acute iritis or middilated and fixed pupils in acute angle-closure glaucoma). Acute visual loss may result from conditions that cause rapid changes in the transparency of these tissues.

Corneal Edema

One cause of sudden opacification of the cornea is corneal edema, which is recognized by a dulling of the normally crisp reflection of incident light off the cornea. The cornea, crystal-clear when healthy, takes on a ground-glass appearance.

The most common cause of corneal edema is increased intraocular pressure. Visual loss accompanying an attack of angle-closure glaucoma (an ocular emergency) is largely the result of corneal edema. (See Slide 22 in Chapter 4.) Chronic damage to the corneal endothelium by dystrophies or following cataract surgery produces corneal edema, but the visual loss has a gradual onset. Any acute infection or inflammation of the cornea (eg, herpes simplex keratitis) may mimic corneal edema.

Hyphema

Blood in the anterior chamber is known as a *hyphema* (see Slide 42 in Chapter 5). Any significant hyphema reduces vision, and a complete hyphema will reduce vision to light perception only. Lesser degrees of hyphema may not affect visual acuity. Most hyphemas are the direct consequence of blunt trauma to a normal eye; however, the presence of abnormal vessels (which occurs with tumors, diabetes, intraocular surgery, and chronic inflammation—all causes of neovascularization) predisposes to hyphema.

Cataract

Most cataracts develop slowly. The rare patient may interpret rapid progression of a cataract as sudden visual loss. Even in a patient with a clear lens, sudden changes in blood sugar or serum electrolytes can alter the hydration of the lens. These changes in lens hydration can result in large fluctuations in refractive error, which may be interpreted by the patient as visual loss. In this situation, acuity may simply be improved with refraction.

Vitreous Hemorrhage

Bleeding into the vitreous reduces vision in the same way that hyphema does: in relation to the amount and location of opaque blood. Large vitreous hemorrhages occur after trauma and in any condition causing retinal neovascularization (eg, diabetes or retinal vein occlusion). In addition, vitreous hemorrhage may accompany subarachnoid hemorrhage and is one cause of visual loss from aneurysms. Vitreous hemorrhage may be difficult to appreciate when viewed with the ophthalmoscope, especially through an undilated pupil. If the red reflex cannot be seen but the lens appears clear, vitreous hemorrhage should be suspected. Diagnosis can be confirmed by an ophthalmologist with slit-lamp examination through a dilated pupil.

Retinal Disease

Retinal detachment, macular disease, and retinal vascular occlusion are all associated with sudden visual loss. However, acute visual loss may develop in any inflammatory process that affects the retina, including infectious chorioretinitis, vasculitides, and idiopathic inflammation. These conditions may be distinguished from other causes of acute visual loss by their ophthalmoscopic findings.

Retinal Detachment

Acute visual loss is a feature of an extensive retinal detachment. Typically, the patient with a retinal detachment (Slide 7) complains of flashing lights followed by large numbers of floaters and then a shade over the vision in one eye. A detachment extensive enough to reduce visual acuity usually produces a relative afferent pupillary defect in the involved eye. The diagnosis is made by ophthalmoscopy through the dilated pupil. The retina appears elevated, sometimes with folds, and the choroidal background is indistinct. However, the findings may not be obvious, and emergency ophthalmologic consultation is indicated.

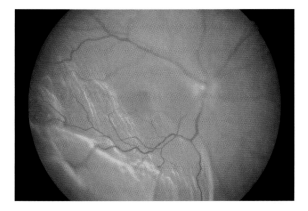

Slide 7   Retinal detachment. A 60° view of the fundus reveals folds of retina extending into the macula inferotemporal to the disc. In this photograph, the focus is on the elevated retina, which renders the disc slightly out of focus.

Macular Disease

Macular disease reduces visual acuity, but unless the disease is extensive, a relative afferent pupillary defect may not be present. Sudden visual loss from macular disease is often an index of bleeding from a neovascular net formed as part of the process of age-related macular degeneration (see Chapter 3). If the visual loss is preceded by metamorphopsia (a defect of central vision in which the shapes of objects appear distorted), the neovascularization may be identified and treated with laser surgery before progression to significant and permanent visual loss occurs.

Retinal Vascular Occlusion

Retinal vascular occlusion is a relatively common cause of sudden visual loss and may be transient or permanent. Transient monocular visual loss due to arterial insufficiency is called *amaurosis fugax* and is a very important symptom. In a patient over age 50, the report of visual loss in one eye lasting for several minutes should lead to investigation of the ipsilateral carotid circulation, looking for an atheroma, which may be the source of emboli that transiently interrupt blood flow to the retina. The evaluation and management of such a patient raises complicated issues, and referral should be made to an ophthalmologist, a neurologist, or a vascular surgeon.

Central Retinal Artery Occlusion   Prolonged interruption of retinal arterial blood flow causes permanent damage to the ganglion cells and other tissue elements. Central retinal artery occlusion (Slide 8) is manifested as a sudden, painless, and often complete visual loss. The ophthalmoscopic appearance depends on how soon after the visual loss the fundus is seen. Within minutes to hours, the only findings may be vascular stasis: narrowing of arterial blood columns and interruption of venous blood columns with the appearance of "boxcarring" as rows of corpuscles are separated by clear intervals.

Some hours after a central retinal artery occlusion, the inner layer of the retina becomes opalescent. The loss of the normal transparency of the retina is most visible ophthalmoscopically where the retina is thickest

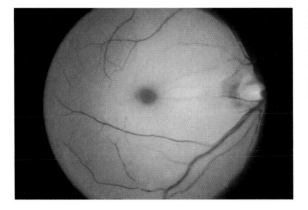

Slide 8   Central retinal artery occlusion. The retina is opaque, except for the relatively thin area within the macula, producing the "cherry-red spot."

around the fovea. In the fovea itself, the inner layers are attenuated. Pallor of the perifoveal retina stands in contrast to the normal color of the fovea, causing the characteristic "cherry-red spot" of central retinal artery occlusion. A chronic cherry-red spot is also a feature of storage diseases, such as Tay-Sachs disease and some variants of Niemann-Pick disease, in which the ganglion cells become opalescent because of the deposition of intermediate metabolites.

The optic disc, which is supplied by other branches of the ophthalmic artery, does not swell unless the occlusion is in the ophthalmic or carotid artery, proximal to the origin of the central retinal artery or in the small vessels supplying the disc. The peculiarities of the eye's vascular supply also can explain the possible preservation of some vision in the presence of a complete central retinal artery occlusion. If part of the retina derives its blood supply from the choroidal circulation via a cilioretinal artery, its function is spared. After a central retinal artery occlusion, the retinal edema slowly resolves and the death of the ganglion cells and their axons leads to optic atrophy. Months later, the characteristic ophthalmoscopic appearance is a pale disc in a blind eye.

When ophthalmoscopy shows the diagnosis of an acute central retinal artery occlusion, immediate treatment is warranted unless circulation has already been restored spontaneously. *This is a true ophthalmic emergency;* restoration of blood flow may preserve vision if the occlusion is only a few hours old. Instances are reported in which vision has returned after treatment of an occlusion that has been present for several days. In a blind eye, there is little to lose by aggressive measures, and an ophthalmologist's advice should be obtained as quickly as possible.

As an emergency measure, the primary care physician may wish to compress the eye with the heel of the hand, pressing firmly for 10 seconds and then releasing for 10 seconds over a period of approximately 5 minutes. The sudden rise and fall in intraocular pressure could serve to dislodge a small embolus in the central retinal artery and restore circulation before the retinal tissues sustain irreversible damage. An ophthalmologist might employ more vigorous and invasive techniques, including retrobulbar injection of an anesthetic and paracentesis of the anterior chamber.

Branch Retinal Artery Occlusion   When only a branch of the central retinal artery is occluded, only part of the retina opacifies and vision is only partially lost. A branch retinal artery occlusion is more likely to be the result of an embolus than is a central retinal artery occlusion, and a source should be sought. If visual acuity is affected, attempts should be made to dislodge the embolus by ocular massage, as discussed above.

Central Retinal Vein Occlusion   The ophthalmoscopic picture of disc swelling, venous engorgement, cotton-wool spots (which appear as small white patches on the retina), and diffuse retinal hemorrhages indicates a central retinal vein occlusion (Slide 9). Loss of vision may be severe, although the onset is generally subacute, unlike the dramatic sudden blindness of a central retinal artery occlusion. The fundus picture is so striking that the description "blood and thunder" is sometimes applied.

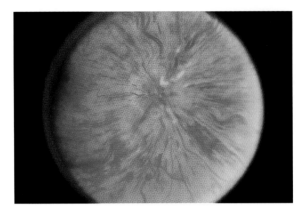

Slide 9 Central retinal vein occlusion. Dilated and tortuous veins, flame-shaped hemorrhages, and cotton-wool spots characterize this condition.

Despite its dramatic appearance, there is no generally accepted acute management, and a central retinal vein occlusion is not a true ophthalmic emergency.

A central retinal vein occlusion is most often encountered in older patients with hypertension and arteriosclerotic vascular disease. Carotid artery occlusion may produce a similar but milder fundus picture. In rare cases, diseases that alter blood viscosity—such as polycythemia vera, sickle-cell disease, and lymphoma-leukemia—induce a central retinal vein occlusion.

The acute hemorrhages and disc swelling resolve with time; however, they may be followed by the development of shunt vessels from the retinal to the choroidal circulation and by ocular neovascularization. The patient with a central retinal vein occlusion needs a general medical evaluation and followup by an ophthalmologist, who may be able to prevent the late complication of neovascular glaucoma by performing laser photocoagulation surgery of the ischemic retina.

Optic Nerve Disease

Conditions affecting the optic nerve can often result in acute visual loss. Although the optic nerve head may or may not appear normal initially by ophthalmoscopy, pupillary responses are usually abnormal in unilateral disease.

Optic Neuritis

Optic neuritis is an inflammation of the optic nerve that is usually idiopathic but may be associated with multiple sclerosis in a significant number of cases. Reduced visual acuity and a relative afferent pupillary defect are regular features of optic neuritis. The optic disc appears hyperemic and swollen. The prognosis for the return of vision after a single attack of optic neuritis is good. Patients with suspected optic neuritis should be referred to an ophthalmologist for further evaluation. Certain patients with optic neuritis may benefit from high-dose intravenous corticosteroids.

Retrobulbar Optic Neuritis

A young adult who is experiencing a monocular loss of vision that has developed over hours to days and that is often accompanied by pain on movement of the eye but who shows no abnormalities on ophthalmoscopic examination probably has retrobulbar optic neuritis. Again, vision is poor and an afferent pupillary defect is present. Included in the differential diagnosis of retrobulbar optic neuritis is compressive optic neuropathy, which can appear as acute visual loss. The pattern of visual field loss may point to a noninflammatory cause, for example, by a finding of visual field loss in the other eye. Computed tomography or magnetic resonance imaging of the orbits and chiasmal region will identify most compressive lesions, which are potentially treatable with surgery.

Papillitis and Papilledema

Like retrobulbar optic neuritis, papillitis (Slide 10) is a subtype of optic neuritis. Specifically, papillitis is an inflammation of the optic disc, or papilla. Papilledema (Slide 11), on the other hand, refers to swelling of the optic disc from increased intracranial pressure; both optic discs are affected. In optic neuritis (either retrobulbar neuritis or papillitis), vision is usually (but not always) significantly decreased and examination of the

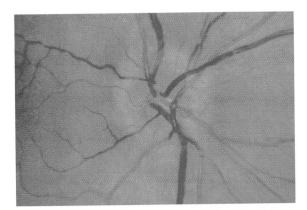

Slide 10   Papillitis. The disc is swollen, with blurred disc margins. In papillitis, the disc is hyperemic, rather than pale as in ischemic optic neuropathy. Papillitis is usually unilateral. Bilateral papillitis can be differentiated from papilledema based on decreased visual acuity in papillitis.

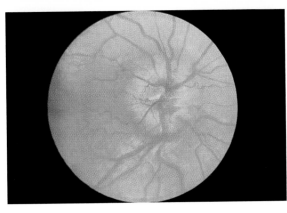

Slide 11   Papilledema. The optic disc is elevated and the margins are indistinct. There is microvascular congestion on the disc, the retinal veins are dilated, and flame-shaped hemorrhages are present. The appearance in the other eye should be similar.

pupils will reveal a relative afferent pupillary defect. In papilledema, the visual acuity and the pupillary reflexes are usually normal.

Some patients with acute papilledema complain of momentary blurring or transient obscurations of vision. Although chronic papilledema may lead to loss of vision, most patients with acute papilledema suffer only minor alterations in vision.

Ischemic Optic Neuropathy

Swelling of the disc and visual loss in an older adult are likely to represent a vascular event rather than inflammation. Ischemic optic neuropathy (Slide 12) is a vascular disorder that presents as a pale, swollen disc, often accompanied by splinter hemorrhages and loss of visual acuity and visual field. The field loss with ischemic neuropathy is often predominantly in the superior or inferior field, a pattern known as *altitudinal*.

Giant-Cell Arteritis

The development of acute ischemic optic neuropathy in a patient over age 60 raises the possibility of giant-cell, or temporal, arteritis. When this systemic arteritis is present, there are often associated complaints of malaise, headache, fever, weight loss, pain and tenderness of muscles and joints (polymyalgia rheumatica), scalp tenderness or discomfort when combing the hair, and a virtually pathognomonic pain in the jaws on chewing, termed *jaw claudication*. Ocular complaints may include sudden visual loss and diplopia (double vision).

Even in an otherwise asymptomatic elderly patient who has ischemic optic neuropathy (or, for that matter, a central retinal artery occlusion or an unexplained ophthalmoplegia, a paresis of extraocular movement), a sedimentation rate should be obtained immediately. Many elderly persons with giant-cell arteritis have markedly elevated sedimentation rates, to greater than 60 mm per hour. If the sedimentation rate is elevated or if there are other symptoms or signs of giant-cell arteritis, treatment with high-dose systemic corticosteroids is mandatory unless there is a very strong contraindication to their use. This course of treatment may preserve

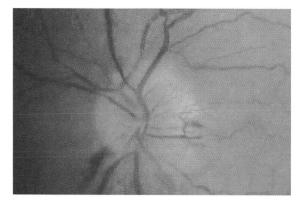

Slide 12 Ischemic optic neuropathy. This figure shows pale swelling of the optic disc, with associated flame-shaped hemorrhages.

vision in the remaining eye and prevent vascular occlusions elsewhere that would cause stroke or myocardial infarction. *Immediate referral to an ophthalmologist is indicated if giant-cell arteritis is a strong diagnostic possibility.* Biopsy of the temporal artery may demonstrate pathologic changes that confirm the diagnosis: giant cells, fragmentation of the elastica with surrounding chronic inflammation, and occlusion of the vessel.

If no systemic arteritis is demonstrated, there is no clear evidence that systemic corticosteroids benefit patients with ischemic optic neuropathy. Unfortunately, there is an approximately 40% chance that the other eye will become involved with nonarteritic ischemic optic neuropathy, with or without treatment.

Trauma

Trauma is another potential cause of visual loss due to involvement of the optic nerve (traumatic optic neuropathy). Apparently, in a small number of cases, concussive head trauma shears the vascular supply to the optic nerve, producing blindness. Surgical decompression of the optic canal may be undertaken in selected cases.

Visual Pathway Disorders

Hemianopia

The cerebral visual pathways are susceptible to involvement by vascular events or tumors. In older persons, a homonymous hemianopia, defined as loss of vision on one side of both visual fields, may result from occlusion of one of the posterior cerebral arteries with infarction of the occipital lobe. Other vascular events occurring in the middle cerebral artery distribution also may produce a hemianopia, but usually other neurologic signs are prominent. Almost any patient with a hemianopia warrants examination by cerebral computed tomography or magnetic resonance imaging to localize and identify the cause. See Chapter 7 for further information about hemianopic visual field loss.

Cortical Blindness

Much rarer than a hemianopia is extensive bilateral damage to the cerebral visual pathways resulting in complete loss of vision. This condition is referred to variously as *cortical, central*, or *cerebral blindness*. Because the pathways serving the pupillary light reflex separate from those carrying visual information at the level of the optic tracts, a patient who is cortically blind has normal pupillary reactions. This finding, along with a normal fundus on ophthalmoscopic examination, helps make the diagnosis of cortical blindness. Most patients with cortical blindness either improve or will die due to severe neurologic damage. Transient cortical blindness has been observed in children after subconcussive head trauma.

Functional Disorders

The adjective *functional* is used in preference to *hysterical* or *malingering* to describe visual loss without organic basis. Often the diagnosis is apparent because the examination produces results incompatible with organic blindness. For example, the patient who reports complete blindness in one eye and normal vision in the other but has normal stereopsis and no relative afferent pupillary defect most likely has a functional disorder. In other patients, sophisticated ophthalmologic examinations may be necessary to make an accurate diagnosis.

Acute Discovery of Chronic Visual Loss

A surprising number of cases of chronic visual loss turn up as acute discoveries. Because the eyes usually function together, this sudden discovery of what has actually been an ongoing problem is most likely to occur when the vision in one eye is normal. A person who claims acute visual loss in one eye but has advanced optic atrophy must have had a prolonged but unrecognized problem. In doubtful cases, it is desirable to obtain records of previous formal eye examinations before accepting visual loss as an acute event and proceeding with expensive or invasive workups.

Points to Remember

1. Early, accurate diagnosis and timely treatment are critical to a positive visual outcome in cases of acute visual loss.
2. Patient ocular history, including timing, tempo, and unilaterality or bilaterality of visual loss, as well as medical history and prior visual acuity, are important to accurate diagnosis.
3. Pupillary responses, visual field testing, and ophthalmoscopy are particularly valuable in determining the causes of acute visual loss.
4. The following conditions require emergency measures and referral: acute angle-closure glaucoma; retinal detachment; acute central retinal artery occlusion; ischemic optic neuropathy if suspected to be related to giant-cell arteritis.

Sample Problems

1. A 58-year-old woman complains of a sudden shower of dust-like particles floating before her right eye. You record VA as 20/20 in each eye. Upon dilated ophthalmoscopy, you see a normal fundus. Your diagnosis is of a possible retinal tear, with the danger of retinal detachment. What is your course of action?

   Answer: Prompt ophthalmologic consultation. A sudden shower of floaters may indicate red blood cells in the vitreous due to a retinal tear. Floaters may be visible to the patient but not to the ophthalmoscopist.

Because the retina has no sensitivity to pain and is, in fact, limited to the sensation of light, the patient may report flashes of light as the retina tears or detaches. Retinal tears usually are located in the far periphery of the retina and may easily elude detection. Symptoms alone indicate the need for referral.

2. A 67-year-old man experienced sudden loss of vision in the left eye 3 hours ago. You record VA as OD 20/20 and OS no light perception. The right pupil responds to light directly but not consensually. The left pupil responds to light consensually but not directly. Dilated fundus examination of the right eye is normal. The left eye shows a white, opacified retina, a cherry-red spot in the macula, and sluggish retinal circulation. You diagnose a central retinal artery occlusion. What is the proper management?

   Answer: You use the heel of your hand to apply pressure to the affected eye, pressing and releasing several times, in the hope that the induced alterations of intraocular pressure may dislodge an embolus. You seek ophthalmologic consultation and undertake a prompt search for the cause of this vascular event.

   Because the retina is neural tissue and survives complete circulatory deprivation poorly, the prognosis for recovery of useful vision in the affected eye is not good. Probably as important is the detection of underlying disease (such as giant-cell arteritis) or a site of embolus formation (such as carotid atheroma) that might lead to future vascular occlusions.

3. A 78-year-old man has recently noticed poor vision in the right eye. He thinks the onset was rather sudden. He has been otherwise healthy but has lost 5 pounds over the last month and thinks he has "less energy." He also has noticed a headache on the right side over the last several days. Your examination reveals a visual acuity of 20/70 on the right and 20/30 on the left. The right pupil seems suspicious for an afferent pupillary defect but is difficult to interpret. The optic nerve looks swollen on the right. What is your course of action?

   Answer: The patient has giant-cell arteritis but does not have all of the classic symptoms and signs. Your index of suspicion should be high in this patient because of his reduced vision, possible afferent pupillary defect, headache, and swollen optic nerve. Obtain a STAT sedimentation rate and refer the patient to an ophthalmologist immediately. High-dose systemic corticosteroids may be needed to preserve vision and prevent other systemic complications.

Annotated Resources

Beck RW, Cleary PA, Trobe JD, et al: The effect of corticosteroids for acute optic neuritis on the subsequent development of multiple sclerosis. The Optic Neuritis Study Group. *N Engl J Med* 1993;329:1764–1769. In this multicenter randomized controlled clinical trial involving 389 patients without known multiple sclerosis, short-term high-dose IV corticosteroid administration appeared to reduce the rate of development of the disease over a 2-year period.

Boghen DR, Glaser JA: Ischemic optic neuritis: the clinical profile and natural history. *Brain* 1975;98:689–708. This article clearly distinguishes the different types (arteritic vs nonarteritic ischemic optic neuritis) and gives a good discussion of the natural history of these several conditions.

Gutman FA: Evaluation of a patient with central retinal vein occlusion. *Ophthalmology* 1983;90:481–483. One of several articles in the same volume of this journal outlining the diagnosis, evaluation, and management of central retinal vein occlusions.

Hurwitz BJ, Heyman A, Wilkinson WE, et al: Comparison of amaurosis fugax and transient cerebral ischemia: a prospective clinical and arteriographic study. *Ann Neurol* 1985;18:698–704. This series of over 300 patients with amaurosis fugax or transient cerebral ischemic attacks is part of a large literature on the subject, but one of the few prospective studies. Two thirds of middle-aged or elderly patients with amaurosis fugax had operable carotid lesions.

Miller NR, Newman N: *Walsh & Hoyt's Clinical Neuro-Ophthalmology*. 5th ed. Baltimore: Williams & Wilkins; 1997. The second volume of this excellent four-volume set provides an extensive discussion of disorders of the optic nerve.

Ravits J, Seybold ME: Transient monocular visual loss from narrow-angle glaucoma. *Arch Neurol* 1984;41:991–993. Three patients with intermittent angle-closure glaucoma had their transient visual loss attributed to other causes until glaucoma was considered.

Rizzo JF, Lessell S: Risk of developing multiple sclerosis after uncomplicated optic neuritis. *Neurology* 1988;38:185–190. A good discussion of the factors to be considered before assigning an episode of optic neuritis to a demyelinating etiology.

Savino PJ, Glaser JS, Cassady J: Retinal stroke: is the patient at risk? *Arch Ophthalmol* 1977;95:1185–1189. A review of different forms of retinal artery occlusion, with recommendations regarding causes and approaches.

Trobe JD: *The Physician's Guide to Eye Care*. San Francisco: American Academy of Ophthalmology; 1993. A brief but comprehensive resource covering the principal clinical ophthalmic problems that nonophthalmologist physicians are likely to encounter, organized for practical use by practitioners.

Chapter 3

Chronic Visual Loss

Objectives

As a primary care physician, you should be familiar with the major causes of chronic, slowly progressive visual loss in an adult patient—namely, glaucoma, cataract, and macular degeneration—and be able to identify the basic characteristics of each. (See also Chapter 8 for a discussion of diabetic retinopathy, another important cause of chronic visual loss.) In addition, you should be able to evaluate the nerve head, classifying it as normal, glaucomatous, or abnormal but nonglaucomatous. You also should be able to evaluate the clarity of the lens as well as the function and appearance of the macula.

To achieve these objectives, you should learn

- To recognize those characteristics of the optic disc useful in determining whether a given disc is normal or abnormal
- To recognize a cataract and to determine its approximate potential effect on the patient's vision
- To determine whether a cataract is the only cause of a patient's visual decrease
- To examine the macula with the ophthalmoscope and recognize the signs and symptoms of maculopathy

Glaucoma

Relevance

Glaucoma is a significant cause of blindness in the United States and is the most frequent cause of blindness among African Americans. If glaucoma is detected early and treated medically or surgically, blindness can be prevented. Most patients with early glaucoma are asymptomatic. The great majority of patients lack pain, ocular inflammation, or halos (luminous or colored rings seen around lights). Much peripheral vision can be lost before the patient notices visual disability.

Glaucoma is usually insidious because symptoms and noticeable visual field defects occur late in the disease. Visual field defects are characterized by arcuate-shaped scotomas (areas of reduced or absent vision) and a contraction of the peripheral field, usually sparing the central vision until late in the disease process. Detection in the early asymptomatic stage requires an active effort. The early detection of glaucoma is important because blindness can usually be prevented if glaucoma is treated adequately and if treatment is begun in time.

Because glaucoma usually involves elevation of intraocular pressure above the statistically normal range, routine measurement of the pressure is a valuable means of screening for glaucoma. Prolonged elevation of intraocular pressure can lead to optic nerve damage, but in some cases, glaucomatous optic nerve changes are evident despite an apparently normal pressure. Therefore, examination of the optic nerve is another way to detect glaucoma. Other disorders, such as brain tumor, can also cause changes in the optic nerve, making the ability to recognize abnormalities of the optic nerve important in and of itself.

Basic Information

Intraocular Pressure

Within the eye is a mechanism for the continuous production and drainage of fluid. This fluid, called *aqueous humor*, is produced by the ciliary body of the eye. Aqueous humor flows through the pupil into the anterior chamber, where it is drained through the trabecular meshwork to Schlemm's canal (Figure 3.1), and onward to the venous system. Because of some resistance to the flow of aqueous through the trabeculum and Schlemm's canal, pressure is created in the eye. All eyes have an internal pressure.

Intraocular pressure is largely dependent on the ease of flow through the trabeculum and Schlemm's canal. The greater the resistance to flow, the higher the pressure in the eye. Although the eye contains several compartments within it, for purposes of pressure it can be considered a single closed space. Thus, the pressure exerted within the eye is equal over the entire wall of the eye. Most normal eyes have an intraocular pressure (IOP) of 21 mm Hg or less.

In the common, insidious form of glaucoma, the chamber angle remains open. Accordingly, this form of glaucoma is called *open-angle glaucoma*. In rare instances, the trabeculum can become suddenly and completely occluded by iris tissue. This causes an abrupt rise in intraocular pressure known as *acute angle-closure glaucoma* (see Slide 22 in Chapter 4) and constitutes an ocular emergency. The abrupt rise in pressure causes symptoms not found in the insidious form of glaucoma, including pain, nausea, and the visualization of colored halos or rainbows around light. An acute attack of angle closure usually produces a red, teary eye with a hazy cornea and a fixed, middilated pupil. The eye feels extremely firm to palpation in most cases.

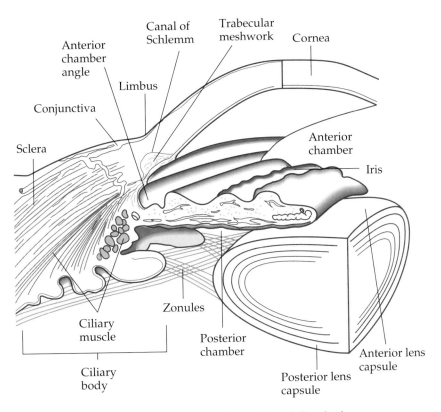

Figure 3.1   Cross-section of anterior chamber angle and ciliary body.

Optic Nerve

The optic nerve is composed of more than 1.2 million nerve fibers. These nerve fibers originate in the ganglion cells of the retina, gather in a bundle as the optic nerve, and carry visual information to the brain. An interruption of these nerve fibers results in damage to vision.

The optic nerve can be seen at its origin by using the ophthalmoscope. At the point of origin, the nerve is called the *optic disc*. The optic disc often has a small depression in it called the *cup of the optic disc*. The size of the cup in normal eyes can vary with the individual. A complete description of the optic disc appears in Chapter 1.

Relationship of IOP and Optic Nerve

Intraocular pressure is exerted on all walls of the eye, including the optic nerve and its blood vessels. The optic nerve is supplied with blood via branches of the ophthalmic artery, itself a branch of the internal carotid artery. If pressure in the eye is too high, the result may be that blood is prevented from adequately perfusing the optic nerve. If prolonged, this deficiency can damage the nerve. (Mechanical injury can also cause optic nerve damage; see "Optic Atrophy" in Chapter 7.)

Damage to the optic nerve results in visual field loss. Such loss is selective but can become severe and even total over time. Detection of glaucomatous visual loss is accomplished by visual field testing. Visual acuity usually does not suffer initially. Measurement of intraocular pressure and evaluation of optic nerve appearance can detect potential and actual damage so that proper evaluation and treatment can be initiated.

When to Examine

Ophthalmoscopy should be part of every comprehensive eye examination. Particular attention should be given to patients who are predisposed to glaucoma, such as elderly individuals or those with a family history of glaucoma. The American Academy of Ophthalmology recommends a glaucoma screening every 2 to 4 years past age 40, as the incidence of the disease increases with age. Because African-Americans have an even greater risk for development of glaucoma, those between ages 20 and 39 should additionally be screened every 3 to 5 years.

How to Examine

Palpation can detect only very hard and very soft eyes; it is totally unreliable in the range of the most common glaucomatous intraocular pressures. Intraocular pressure is best measured via tonometry, which may be performed in any of several ways. Indentation, or Schiøtz, tonometry involves an inexpensive instrument that is simple to use. However, hand-held applanation tonometers are available and give much more reliable readings. Although more costly, these are also easy to use and require no special patient positioning. Detailed information on various methods of tonometry appears in Chapter 1. The technique of direct ophthalmoscopy, also described in Chapter 1, is particularly useful in assessing the state of the optic disc.

An ophthalmologist evaluating a patient with suspected glaucoma will usually perform perimetry to formally evaluate the visual field. The ophthalmologist also may examine the anterior chamber angle structures using a special contact lens on the topically anesthetized cornea, a technique called *gonioscopy*.

How to Interpret
the Findings

The appearance of the optic disc can be described generally in terms of its color and of the size of its physiologic cup (a recognizable central depression within the optic disc). The color of the optic nerve can be important in determining atrophy of the nerve that is due to glaucoma or other causes.

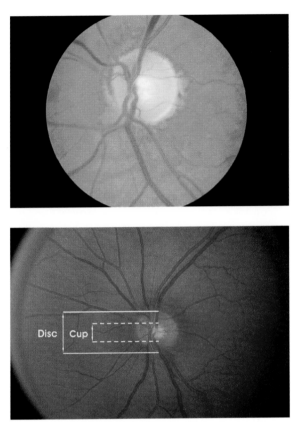

Slide 13 Temporal pallor of the optic nerve. Diseases that damage optic nerve fibers may result in temporal pallor of the optic nerve. Note the normal nerve color present only on the nasal aspect of the disc.

Slide 14 Cup:disc ratio. In this nondiseased optic disc, the cup is less than one half the diameter of the disc, indicating absent or low level of suspicion of glaucoma.

Temporal pallor of the optic nerve (Slide 13) can occur as a result of diseases that damage the nerve fibers, such as brain tumors or optic nerve inflammation, or in conjunction with glaucomatous cupping.

The term *glaucomatous cupping* refers to an increase in the size of the optic cup relative to the optic disc that occurs in glaucoma. This so-called cup:disc ratio is determined by comparing the diameter of the disc to that of the cup (Slide 14). The larger the cup, the greater the probability of a glaucomatous optic nerve. A cup measuring one half the size of the disc or larger—a cup:disc ratio of 0.5 or more—raises suspicion of glaucoma (Slide 15). A large cup should be suspected if central pallor of the disc is prominent. Because the cup is a depressed area of the disc, retinal vessels passing over the disc are seen to bend at the edge of the cup, a useful sign in evaluating cup size. Vessel displacement, then, as well as disc color, should be evaluated in determining the size of the cup (Slide 16).

The optic discs generally should appear symmetric between the eyes. Discs that exhibit asymmetric cup:disc ratios should arouse suspicion. In some cases, edema of the optic disc may be present (called *papilledema* when caused by elevated intracranial pressure), and the cup may be reduced or obliterated (see Slide 11 in Chapter 2).

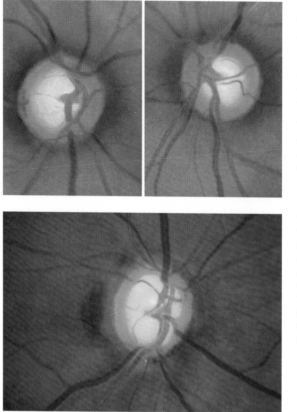

Slide 15   Glaucomatous cupping. The left side shows a cup:disc ratio of 0.9 (high level of glaucoma suspicion) and the right side shows a cup:disc ratio of 0.7 (moderate level of glaucoma suspicion). The asymmetry of the cup:disc ratios here also raises suspicion of glaucoma.

Slide 16   Glaucomatous optic atrophy. Optic nerve cupping is increased vertically, with a cup:disc ratio of 0.8. Cupping is apparent at the point where the vessels disappear over the edge of the attenuated rim.

Management or Referral

Table 3.1 provides a convenient method of analyzing a patient's level of glaucoma risk. A moderate or high level of glaucoma risk warrants referral to an ophthalmologist for further evaluation. In addition, any patient who has one or more of the following conditions should be referred to an ophthalmologist:

- Intraocular pressure over 21 mm Hg
- Intraocular pressure not elevated, but a difference of 5 mm Hg or more between the eyes
- An optic cup diameter one half or more of the disc diameter (ie, a cup:disc ratio of 0.5 or greater)
- One cup significantly larger in one eye than in the other eye
- Symptoms of acute glaucoma (refer immediately; see Slide 22 in Chapter 4)

For a discussion of systemic side effects of topically administered drugs used in the treatment of glaucoma, see Chapter 9.

Table 3.1   Glaucoma Risk Factor Analysis

History-Based Risk Factor Weights

Variable*	Category	Weight
Age	<50 years	0
	50–64 years	1
	65–74 years	2
	>75 years	3
Race	Caucasian/other	0
	African-American	2
Family History of Glaucoma	Negative or positive in non–first-degree relatives	0
	Positive for parents	1
	Positive for siblings	2
Last Complete Eye Examination	Within past 2 years	0
	2–5 years ago	1
	>5 years ago	2

*Other historical variables, such as high myopia or hyperopia, systemic hypertension, corticosteroid use, and perhaps diabetes, are not strong enough to be assigned a weight but may be considered in the overall assessment of glaucoma risk.

Level of Glaucoma Risk	Weighting Score
High	4 or greater (referral advisable)
Moderate	3 (referral advisable)
Low	2 or less

Cataract

Relevance

Cataract may occur as a congenital or genetic anomaly, as a result of various diseases, or with increasing age. Some degree of cataract formation is to be expected in all persons over age 70. In fact, age-related cataract occurs in about 50% of people between ages 65 and 74 and in about 70% of those over 75. Cataract is the most common cause of decreased vision (not correctable with glasses) in the United States. However, it is one of the most successfully treated conditions in all of surgery. Approximately 1.4 million cataract extractions are done each year in the United States, usually with

implantation of an intraocular lens. If an implant is not used, visual rehabilitation is still possible with a contact lens or thick (aphakic) eyeglasses.

It is important to be certain that visual loss is explained fully by cataract
and not by other causes, such as glaucoma, macular degeneration, or diabetic retinopathy. Cataract may coexist with these conditions, making
assessment more difficult.

Basic Information

Lens

The crystalline lens focuses a clear image on the retina. The lens is suspended by thin filamentous zonules from the ciliary body between the iris
anteriorly and the vitreous humor posteriorly. Contraction of the ciliary
muscle permits focusing of the lens. The lens is enclosed in a capsule of
transparent elastic basement membrane. The capsule encloses the cortex
and the nucleus of the lens as well as a single anterior layer of cuboidal
epithelium. The lens has no innervation or blood supply. Nourishment
comes from the aqueous fluid and the vitreous.

The normal lens continues to grow throughout life. The epithelial cells
continue to produce new cortical lens fibers, yielding a slow increase in
size, weight, and density over the years. The normal lens consists of 35%
protein by mass. The percentage of insoluble protein increases as the lens
ages and as a cataract develops.

Cataract

A cataract is any opacity or discoloration of the lens, whether a small, local
opacity or the complete loss of transparency. Clinically, the term *cataract* is
usually reserved for opacities that affect visual acuity because many normal lenses have small, visually insignificant opacities.

A cataract is described in terms of the zones of the lens involved in the
opacity. These zones of opacity may be subcapsular, cortical, or nuclear
and may be anterior or posterior in location. In addition to opacification of
the nucleus and cortex, there may be a yellow or amber color change to the
lens. A cataract also can be described in terms of its stage of development.
A cataract with a clear cortex remaining is immature (Slide 17). A mature
cataract (Slide 18) has a totally opacified cortex.

The most common cause of cataract is age-related change. Other
causative factors include trauma, inflammation, metabolic and nutritional
defects, and radiation damage. Cataracts may develop very slowly over the
years or may progress rapidly, depending on the cause and type of cataract.

Symptoms of Cataract

Patients may first notice image blur as the lens loses its ability to resolve
separate and distinct objects. Patients are first aware of a disturbance of
vision, then a diminution, and finally a failure of vision. The degree of
visual disability caused by a cataract depends on the size and location of

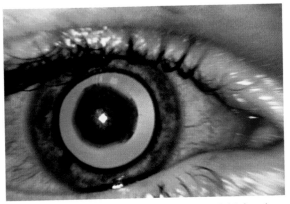

Slide 17 Immature cataract. The nucleus of this lens is opaque (nuclear cataract), while the cortical layers remain clear. The opacity appears as a dark shadow against the red reflex. This particular cataract, which is congenital, will obstruct vision more when the pupil is small than when it is dilated, as shown here.

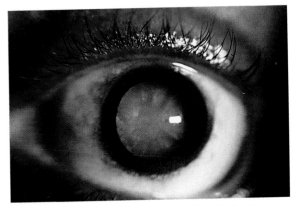

Slide 18 Mature cataract. A cataract is called *mature* when the lens is totally opacified. A red reflex cannot be obtained; the pupil appears white. The radial spokes in this figure reflect variations in density of the radially arranged fibers in the cortical layers of the lens. Light still reaching the retina is totally diffused and will allow the perception of light but not form.

the opacity. Axial opacities—affecting the nucleus or central subcapsular areas (see Slide 17)—cause much more disabling visual loss than do peripheral opacities.

Patients with nuclear sclerosis may develop increasing lenticular (ie, referring to the crystalline lens) myopia because of the increased refractive power of the denser nucleus. As the size of the cataract increases, patients become progressively more myopic. Patients may find they can read without the glasses normally required, a phenomenon often called *second sight*. Patients may note monocular double or multiple images, due to irregular refraction within the lens.

Patients with posterior subcapsular cataracts may note a relatively rapid decrease in vision, with glare as well as image blur and distortion. This type of cataract is frequently associated with metabolic causes such as diabetes mellitus and corticosteroid use.

With enough time, all cataracts will lead to a generalized impairment of vision. The degree of impairment may vary from day to day. With yellowing of the lens nucleus, objects appear browner or yellower to the patient than they actually are.

When to Examine

A patient with decreasing vision requires examination to determine the cause of the visual decrease. In testing for the presence of cataract, it is also important to attempt to demonstrate that the retina and optic nerve are healthy and that the visual decrease is due to lens changes only or primarily.

If the lens is densely cataractous, the ophthalmoscope will not provide a view of the fundus through the opacity. In this situation, the risk of overlooking retinal or other disease conditions exists, as does the risk of performing surgery for cataract without the assurance that vision loss is due primarily to lens changes. Therefore, to detect fundus changes early, ophthalmoscopic examination should be part of every physical examination. Special attention is given to the macula when a patient reports difficulty with near work, blurred vision, or metamorphopsia (ie, a wavy distortion of central vision).

How to Examine

The following examination methods are particularly helpful in determining whether visual loss is attributable to cataract, to some other cause, or to a combination of causes:

- **Visual acuity**   The first step in any evaluation of visual decrease is the measurement of visual acuity. Refer to Chapter 1 for details.
- **Pupillary responses**   Chapter 7 describes how to perform a basic pupillary examination and provides details on the neurologic implications of pupillary responses. Even an advanced cataract would not produce a relative afferent pupillary defect.
- **Ophthalmoscopy**   The examiner's view into the eye should be about the same as the cataract patient's visual acuity; that is, the cataract should affect the physician's view into the eye through the direct ophthalmoscope to about the same extent as it does the patient's view out of the eye.

How to Interpret the Findings

An early cataract is not visible to the unaided eye. If the cataract becomes very dense, it may appear as a white pupil, or leukocoria. The lens can be evaluated with the ophthalmoscope using a plus-lens setting. The lens opacification with a partial cataract will appear black against the red reflex of the fundus (see Slide 17). Generally, the denser the cataract, the poorer the red reflex and the worse the visual acuity.

In addition to ophthalmoscopy, an ophthalmologist would routinely perform a slit-lamp examination, which provides a magnified, stereoscopic view of the lens and other anterior segment structures.

Management or Referral

It is important not to assign visual loss to cataract before ensuring that other, more serious causes of visual loss have not been overlooked. The decision to refer a patient with cataract should be based in part on whether or not the cataract keeps the patient from doing what he or she wants to do. A cataract can interfere with patients' daily activities of living by limiting their ability to drive safely, read, or participate in sports or other hobbies. Patients with cataract-associated visual loss that negatively affects their daily living may benefit from a surgical procedure of cataract extraction with intraocular lens implantation. After cataract-removal surgery, patients commonly undergo a laser surgical procedure to open an opacified posterior capsule, leading to a popular misconception that a cataract can actually be removed with a laser.

Macular Degeneration

Relevance

In the United States, age-related macular degeneration is the leading cause of irreversible central visual loss (20/200 or worse) among people aged 52 or older. Because certain types of macular degeneration are treated effectively with laser, it is important to recognize this entity and to refer for appropriate care. It is important to distinguish between the possible causes of visual loss, whether cataract (surgically correctable), glaucoma (medically or surgically treatable), or macular degeneration (potentially laser treatable).

Basic Information

Macular Anatomy

The macula is an oval area situated about 2 disc diameters temporal and slightly inferior to the optic disc (see Slide 2 in Chapter 1 for a depiction of the normal fundus). The macula is composed of both rods and cones and is the area responsible for detailed, fine central vision. The central macula

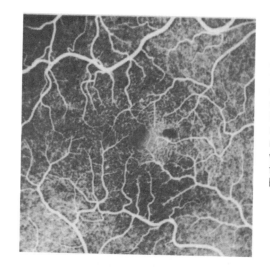

Figure 3.2 Central macula. The central macula is avascular, as demonstrated in this fundus fluorescein angiogram. The central capillary-free zone identifies the foveal region. A small hemorrhage is made more visible against the fluorescein-enhanced background.

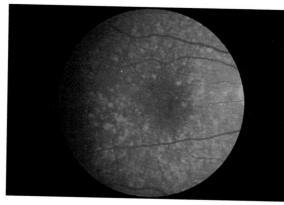

Slide 19 Drusen. Distinct yellow-white lesions may be seen in the posterior pole surrounding the macular area. Although acuity may be normal initially, these lesions can lead to significant visual loss if the central macula becomes involved.

(Figure 3.2) is avascular and appears darker than the surrounding retina. The fovea is an oval depression in the center of the macula. Here, there is a high density of cones but no rods are present. The central depression of the fovea may act like a concave mirror during ophthalmoscopy, producing a light reflection (ie, foveal reflex).

Age-Related Macular Changes

Macular changes due to age include drusen, degenerative changes in the retinal pigment epithelium, and subretinal neovascular membranes.

Drusen are hyaline nodules (or colloid bodies) deposited in Bruch's membrane, which separates the retinal pigment epithelium (the outermost layer of the retina) from the inner choroidal vessels. Drusen may be small and discrete (Slide 19) or larger, with irregular shapes and indistinct edges. Patients with drusen alone tend to have normal or near-normal visual acuity, with minimal metamorphopsia. Drusen may be seen with increasing age, during retinal or choroidal degeneration in disease states, and as a primary dystrophy.

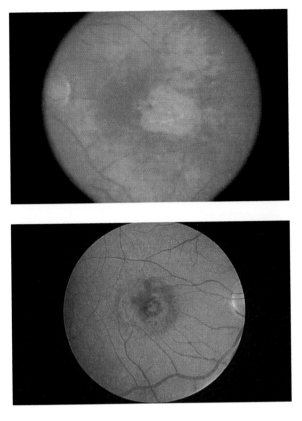

Slide 20 Retinal pigment epithelial atrophy. An irregular area of depigmentation is seen in the macula. The underlying choroidal vasculature is typically more prominent when the pigment epithelium is absent or atrophic.

Slide 21 Subretinal hemorrhage. Age-related macular changes often include subretinal hemorrhage, fibrosis, and pigment epithelial degeneration.

Degenerative changes in the retinal pigment epithelium itself may occur with or without drusen. These degenerative changes are manifested as clumps of hyperpigmentation or depigmented atrophic areas (Slide 20). The effect on visual acuity is variable.

About 20% of eyes with age-related macular degeneration develop subretinal neovascularization. The extension of vessels from the inner choroid layer into the subpigment epithelial space and eventually into the subretinal space means that a defect has developed in Bruch's membrane.

The subretinal neovascular net may be associated with subretinal hemorrhage (Slide 21), fibrosis, pigment epithelial degeneration, and photoreceptor atrophy. A hemorrhage may result in acute visual loss (see Chapter 2). The larger the membrane and the closer to the center of the fovea, the worse the prognosis for good central vision.

Fluorescein angiography, a technique utilized by ophthalmologists, may be necessary to identify neovascularization and is mandatory before considering laser surgery. Intravenous injection of fluorescein dye and subsequent retinal examination or photography help demonstrate the retinal and choroidal vasculature. In contrast to competent retinal veins and arteries, new vessels can be identified because they leak fluorescein dye. In addition, the retinal pigment epithelium acts as a physical and optical barrier to fluorescein, and thus angiography facilitates identification of pigment epithelial defects. Indocyanine green is another dye used to demonstrate new vessels.

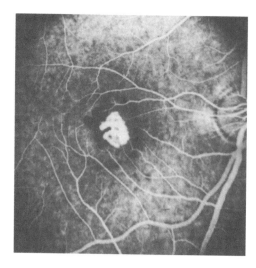

Figure 3.3   Neovascular net. This fluorescein angiogram of the same fundus shown in Slide 21 reveals a subretinal neovascular net, responsible for the subretinal hemorrhage seen in that figure. In this angiogram, the net appears as a white, irregular area of fluorescein leakage.

Compare Slide 21, a fundus photograph depicting a subretinal hemorrhage and other age-related changes, with Figure 3.3, a fundus fluorescein angiogram of the same eye, which reveals neovascularization associated with the hemorrhage. These photographs demonstrate both atrophy and neovascularization.

Age-related changes are almost totally confined to the posterior pole of the eye. Thus, the patient with macular degeneration may have very poor central vision, but will tend to retain functional peripheral vision. Visual aids, such as high-plus magnifiers and telescopic devices, may help the patient. In addition to age, other causes of chronic maculopathy include heredity and metabolic changes.

When to Examine

Any patient with decreasing vision requires examination to determine the cause of the visual decrease. In assessing a patient with decreased or distorted central vision, every effort should be made to examine the macula with the ophthalmoscope. Of course, opacities in the cornea, lens, or vitreous may preclude an adequate view of the macula.

How to Examine

The following techniques are especially helpful in evaluating macular degeneration as the cause of visual decrease or major changes in vision:

- **Visual acuity measurement**   Refer to Chapter 1 for instructions.
- **Amsler grid testing**   Amsler grid testing (Figure 3.4) is a useful method of evaluating the function of the macula. The test is carried out by having the patient look with one eye at a time at a central spot on a page with horizontal and vertical parallel lines making up a square grid pattern. This grid pattern is usually printed in white against a black background. The

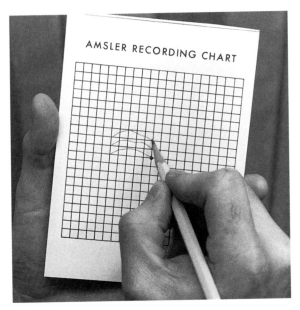

A

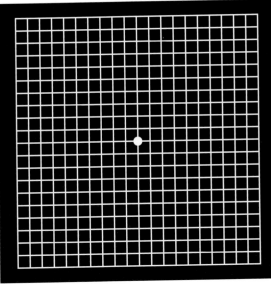

B

Figure 3.4   Amsler grid testing. (**A**) The patient indicates the nature and location of his central field defect by sketching what he perceives on the Amsler grid. (**B**) The typical grid pattern of white lines on a black background.

patient is asked to note irregularities in the lines. Irregularities may be reported as lines that are wavy, seem to bow or bend, appear gray or fuzzy, or are absent in certain areas of the grid, indicating a scotoma.

The straight line, right angle, and square are geometric figures in which the eye can distinguish distortions most easily. With the chart held at a normal reading distance of 30 cm from the eye, the Amsler grid measures 10° on each side of fixation. This allows for an evaluation of 5.36 mm in all directions from the center of the macula (ie, the fovea). Thus, the entire macula is evaluated with this examination.

- **Ophthalmoscopy**   The macular area is studied with the direct ophthalmoscope. Sometimes it is helpful to have the patient look directly into the light of the instrument. Dilation of the pupil may be necessary for adequate examination.
- **Additional studies**   The ophthalmologist may elect to carry out special studies to better evaluate the macula and macular function. Procedures such as stereoscopic slit-lamp examination and fluorescein angiography may be necessary to determine pathologic changes.

How to Interpret the Findings

The appearance of the macula often does not accurately predict the visual acuity. The macula may look more or less involved than the vision indicates. Drusen, areas of decreased or increased pigmentation, subretinal exudate, and hemorrhage or neovascularization are all important signs to check for in an examination of the macula. The absence of the foveal reflex and a mottled appearance of the underlying retinal pigment epithelium are among the early signs of macular disease.

Management or Referral

Any patient who has one or more of the following should be referred to an ophthalmologist:

- A recent onset of decreased visual acuity
- A recent onset of metamorphopsia, or distortion of central vision
- A recent onset of a scotoma, or blind spot
- Any ophthalmoscopic abnormalities in the appearance of the macula, such as drusen, degenerative changes in the retinal pigment epithelium, exudate, or subretinal neovascular membranes

A patient with metamorphopsia may have drusen in the macula only and not be a candidate for laser treatment, but 20% of eyes with age-related macular degeneration develop subretinal neovascularization. Clinical studies have indicated that argon laser photocoagulation of subretinal neovascular membranes that are not too close to the fovea significantly reduces the central visual loss.

The Visually Impaired Patient

Despite medical or surgical therapy, some patients will have a significant residual visual impairment. These patients are candidates for low-vision services and should be referred to an ophthalmologist capable of supplying these services. More than 11 million Americans have a vision impairment that interferes with routine activities; 1.5 million are classified as severely visually handicapped. The use of visual aids will allow many of these patients to continue to function independently. The appropriate and timely intervention by the low-vision specialist is an important part of patients' rehabilitation and should be considered a continuation of their ongoing medical therapy.

Points to Remember

1. Glaucoma should be suspected when ophthalmoscopy reveals either prominent cupping of the optic discs or significant asymmetry of the cup:disc ratio.
2. The primary indication for cataract extraction in most patients is interference with the daily pattern of living rather than reduction of visual acuity to a particular level.
3. Both laser surgery of neovascular membranes and low-vision aids can be helpful to patients with age-related macular degeneration.

Sample Problems

1. During a thorough physical examination of a 38-year-old male patient, you record intraocular pressure of 20 mm Hg in the right eye and 24 mm Hg in the left eye. Based on these findings, which of the following represents a reasonable course of action on your part?
   a. Explain to the patient that he has glaucoma and that you want to recheck his intraocular pressure in 3 months.
   b. Evaluate the optic discs carefully and, if they are normal, recheck the patient in 6 to 12 months.
   c. Refer the patient to an ophthalmologist.
   d. Inquire about a family history of glaucoma and, if there is none, reassure the patient that his intraocular pressure is probably in the upper range of normal.

   Answer: c. Elevated intraocular pressure alone is not a definite indication of glaucoma. It would be correct to tell this patient that his intraocular pressure is slightly elevated on this one occasion. In tonometry screening, it is best to determine the pressure and act accordingly rather than make decisions regarding a definitive diagnosis of glaucoma and a decision on management. Thus, the correct approach in this case is to refer the patient to an ophthalmologist, because pressure of 22 mm Hg or higher is statistically abnormal. The ophthalmologist may decide merely to observe the patient without treatment, but this decision should be left to the ophthalmologist, who should communicate this to the referring physician.

   It is good to know whether the optic discs are normal, but once you find an elevated pressure, your next move should be referral. On the other hand, in situations where you find normal pressure but questionable optic discs, remember that glaucoma still could exist and that referral still may be indicated. Finally, although glaucoma has some hereditary aspects, this should have no bearing in a case in which you find elevated pressure. However, should you have a patient with a strong positive family history of glaucoma, it may be wise to suggest that the patient obtain an ophthalmologist's evaluation despite your finding normal pressure.

2. A retired patient of yours is developing the nuclear sclerotic form of cataract, and his visual acuity has decreased to OD 20/30 and OS 20/40. The only time his vision bothers him is in a dark restaurant, where he has some difficulty reading the menu. Friends have told him about a doctor who will operate with a laser to remove his cataract without risk and who will do it for free. He asks your advice. What do you tell him?
   a. If it's free and he really is a doctor, then go ahead.
   b. Tell him that a laser is not used to remove cataracts, but he should go ahead anyway.
   c. Advise that (1) the indications to remove a cataract are that it endangers the health of the eye or keeps the patient from doing what he needs and wants to do; (2) lasers are not used to remove cataracts; and (3) no surgery is free or without risk. The disability of decreased vision must warrant the risks inherent in surgery.

   Answer: c.

3. A 76-year-old man has noted visual distortion over the past week. His concern increased when he discovered that the distortion was in the right eye only. Straight lines viewed through his left eye remained straight, but they appeared to dip down in the center when viewed with his right eye only. Visual acuity testing revealed 20/50 OD, 20/20 OS.

   A. What further tests will help determine the source of the patient's visual loss?

   Answer: Amsler grid testing will document the patient's symptoms of metamorphopsia. Dilated fundus examination may reveal retinal drusen, retinal hemorrhages secondary to subretinal neovascular membranes, or retinal pigment epithelial atrophy as a manifestation of age-related macular degeneration.

   B. What technique is used by ophthalmologists to identify neovascularization in consideration for laser treatment?

   Answer: Fluorescein angiography is used to document neovascularization.

   C. What percentage of patients with age-related macular degeneration develop subretinal neovascularization?

   Answer: Twenty percent of patients with age-related macular degeneration develop subretinal neovascularization.

Annotated Resources

Jaffe NS, Jaffe MS, Jaffe GF: *Cataract Surgery and Its Complications*. 5th ed. St Louis: CV Mosby Co; 1990. An excellent text covering the contemporary methods of surgical management of cataracts, including phacoemulsification, and the major intraoperative and postoperative complications associated with this surgery.

Macular Photocoagulation Study Group: Argon laser photocoagulation for neovascular maculopathy: three-year results from randomized clinical trials. *Arch Ophthalmol* 1986;104:694–701. The beneficial effects of argon laser photocoagulation are demonstrated in eyes with an extrafoveal choroidal neovascular membrane.

Mangione CM, Phillips RS, Lawrence MG, et al: Improved visual function and attenuation of declines in health-related quality of life after cataract extraction. *Arch Ophthalmol* 1994:112:1419–1425. Improved visual function after cataract surgery was associated with better health-related quality of life, suggesting that age-related declines in health may be attenuated by improvements in visual function.

Shields MB: *Textbook of Glaucoma*. 4th ed. Baltimore: Williams & Wilkins; 1997. An excellent reference covering current medical and surgical therapies of the primary and secondary glaucomas.

Tasman W, Jaeger EA, eds: *Duane's Clinical Ophthalmology*. Philadelphia: JB Lippincott Co; 1996. The section "Diseases of the Lens" in Volume 1 provides basic background material on the anatomy, embryology, and physiology of the lens as well as the pathogenesis of cataract. The section "Glaucoma" in Volume 3 provides information on contemporary concepts about the glaucomas and their treatment. Both basic and sophisticated information is available in this volume. Chapter 23 in Volume 3 covers acquired macular disease, providing current information on age-related macular degeneration.

Trobe JD: *The Physician's Guide to Eye Care*. San Francisco: American Academy of Ophthalmology; 1993. A brief but comprehensive resource covering the principal clinical ophthalmic problems that nonophthalmologist physicians are likely to encounter, organized for practical use by practitioners.

Chapter 4

The Red Eye

Objectives

As a primary care physician, you should be able to determine whether a patient with a red eye requires the prompt attention of an ophthalmologist or whether you can appropriately evaluate and treat the condition.

To achieve this objective, you should learn

- To perform the nine basic diagnostic steps
- To recognize the danger signs of a red eye
- To describe the treatment for those cases you can manage and to recognize the more serious problems that should be referred
- To describe the serious complications of prolonged use of topical anesthetic drops and of corticosteroids

Relevance

A primary care physician frequently encounters patients who complain of a red eye. The condition causing the red eye is often a simple disorder such as a subconjunctival hemorrhage or an infectious conjunctivitis. These conditions either will resolve spontaneously or can be treated easily by the primary care physician. Occasionally, the condition causing a red eye is a more serious disorder, such as intraocular inflammation, corneal inflammation, or acute glaucoma. A patient with one of these vision-threatening conditions requires the immediate attention of an ophthalmologist, whose specialized skills, knowledge, and examining instruments are needed in order to make correct therapeutic decisions.

Basic Information

Red eye refers to hyperemia of the superficially visible vessels of the conjunctiva, episclera, or sclera. Hyperemia, or engorgement of the conjunctival blood vessels, can be caused by disorders of these structures or of adjoining structures, including the cornea, iris, ciliary body, and the ocular adnexa. Specific disorders are discussed in the following section.

Disorders Associated
With a Red Eye

Any patient who complains of a red or painful eye should be examined to diagnose the condition as one of the following:

- **Acute angle-closure glaucoma**   An uncommon form of glaucoma due to sudden and complete occlusion of the anterior chamber angle by iris tissue (Slide 22); serious. The more common chronic open-angle glaucoma causes no redness of the eye. (See Chapter 3 for a discussion of glaucoma.)
- **Iritis or iridocyclitis**   An inflammation of the iris alone or of the iris and ciliary body; often manifested by ciliary flush (Slide 23); serious.
- **Herpes simplex keratitis**   An inflammation of the cornea caused by the herpes simplex virus (Slide 24); common, potentially serious; can lead to corneal ulceration.
- **Conjunctivitis**   Hyperemia of the conjunctival blood vessels (Slide 25); cause may be bacterial, viral, allergic, or irritative; common, often not serious.
- **Episcleritis**   An inflammation (often sectorial) of the episclera, the vascular layer between the conjunctiva and the sclera; uncommon, without discharge, not serious, possibly allergic, occasionally painful.

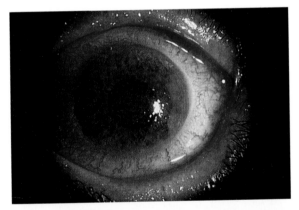

Slide 22   Acute angle-closure glaucoma. The irregular corneal reflection and hazy cornea suggest edema. The pupil is middilated; the iris appears to be displaced anteriorly, with shallowing of the anterior chamber. These findings plus elevated IOP are diagnostic of acute angle-closure glaucoma.

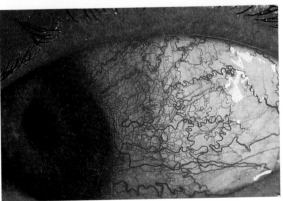

Slide 23   Ciliary flush. Dilated deep conjunctival and episcleral vessels adjacent and circumferential to the corneal limbus cast a violet hue characteristic of ciliary flush and best seen in natural light.

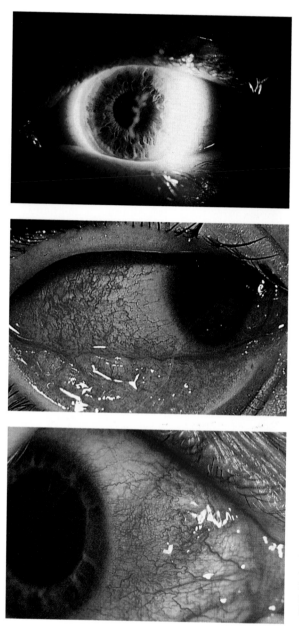

Slide 24 Herpes simplex keratitis. In the center of the cornea is an irregular, dendritic (branch-like) lesion of the corneal epithelium.

Slide 25 Conjunctivitis. The hyperemia seen here is produced by a diffuse dilation of the conjunctival blood vessels. The dilation tends to be less intense in the perilimbal region, in contrast to the perilimbal dilation of deeper vessels characteristic of ciliary flush.

Slide 26 Scleritis. This localized, raised hyperemic lesion is characteristic of scleritis, which is associated with collagen, vascular, and rheumatoid diseases. Episcleritis appears flat, involves more superficial tissue, and is usually not associated with serious systemic disease. The cause of episcleritis may be allergic.

- **Scleritis** An inflammation (localized or diffuse) of the sclera (Slide 26); uncommon, often protracted, usually accompanied by pain; may indicate serious systemic disease such as collagen-vascular disorder; potentially serious to the eye.
- **Adnexal disease** Affects the eyelids, lacrimal apparatus, and orbit; includes dacryocystitis (Slide 27), stye, and blepharitis. Red eye can also occur secondary to lid lesions (such as basal cell carcinoma, squamous cell carcinoma, or molluscum contagiosum), thyroid disease, and vascular lesions in the orbit.

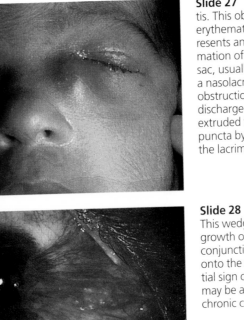

Slide 27 Dacryocystitis. This obvious, raised erythematous mass represents an acute inflammation of the lacrimal sac, usually secondary to a nasolacrimal duct obstruction. A purulent discharge may be extruded from the lid puncta by massage over the lacrimal sac.

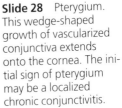

Slide 28 Pterygium. This wedge-shaped growth of vascularized conjunctiva extends onto the cornea. The initial sign of pterygium may be a localized chronic conjunctivitis.

- **Subconjunctival hemorrhage** An accumulation of blood in the potential space between the conjunctiva and the sclera (see Slide 49 in Chapter 5); rarely serious.
- **Pterygium** An abnormal growth consisting of a triangular fold of tissue that advances progressively over the cornea, usually from the nasal side (Slide 28); usually not serious. Localized conjunctival inflammation may be associated with pterygium. Most cases occur in tropical climates. Surgical excision is indicated if the pterygium starts to encroach on the visual axis.
- **Keratoconjunctivitis sicca** A disorder involving the conjunctiva and sclera resulting from lacrimal deficiency; commonly called *dry eyes*; usually not serious.
- **Abrasions and foreign bodies** Hyperemia can occur in response to corneal abrasions or foreign-body injury.
- **Secondary to abnormal lid function** Bell's palsy, thyroid ophthalmopathy, or other lesions causing ocular exposure, such as that which occurs in some comatose patients, can result in a red eye; potentially serious.

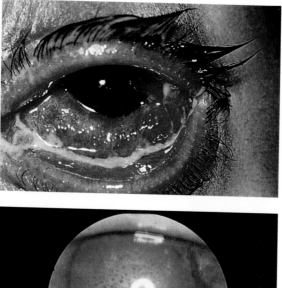

Slide 29 Purulent conjunctivitis. With the lower lid everted, a creamy-white exudate is visible, highlighted by the conjunctival hyperemia.

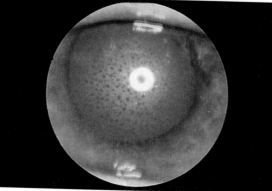

Slide 30 Large keratic precipitates. Multiple gray-white opacities on the back surface of the cornea are seen against the background of the red reflex. These precipitates can result from chronic iridocyclitis.

How to Examine

Nine diagnostic steps are used to evaluate a patient with a red eye:

1. Determine whether the visual acuity is normal or decreased, using a Snellen chart (see Chapter 1).
2. Decide by inspection what pattern of redness is present and whether it is due to subconjunctival hemorrhage, conjunctival hyperemia, ciliary flush, or a combination of these.
3. Detect the presence of conjunctival discharge and categorize it as to amount—profuse or scant—and character—purulent (Slide 29), mucopurulent, or serous.
4. Detect opacities of the cornea, including large keratic precipitates (Slide 30) or irregularities of the corneal surface such as corneal edema (Slide 31), corneal leukoma (a white opacity caused by scar tissue, Slide 32), and irregular corneal reflection (Slide 33). Examination is done using a penlight or transilluminator.
5. Search for disruption of the corneal epithelium by staining the cornea with fluorescein (see Chapter 1).
6. Estimate the depth of the anterior chamber as normal or shallow (see Chapter 1); detect any layered blood or pus, which would indicate either hyphema or hypopyon, respectively. (Compare Slide 34, a corneal ulcer with hypopyon, with hyphema, Slide 42, Chapter 5.)

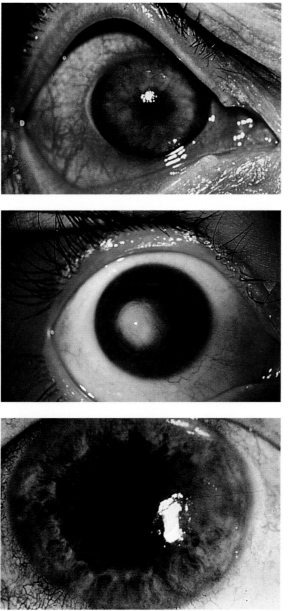

Slide 31 Corneal edema. In this fiery red eye, the normally sharp corneal reflex is replaced by a diffuse, hazy appearance. Iris details are not as clear as in a healthy eye.

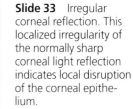

Slide 32 Corneal leukoma. This dense, white corneal scar represents fibrosis secondary to a previous corneal insult, most frequently trauma or infection. Outside the scar, the cornea is clear. If the scar encroaches on the visual axis, acuity may be impaired.

Slide 33 Irregular corneal reflection. This localized irregularity of the normally sharp corneal light reflection indicates local disruption of the corneal epithelium.

7. Detect irregularity of the pupils and determine whether one pupil is larger than the other. Observe the reactivity of the pupils to light to determine whether one pupil is more sluggish than the other or is non-reactive (see Chapters 1 and 7).
8. If elevated intraocular pressure is suspected, as in angle-closure glaucoma, and reliable tonometry is available, then measurement of intraocular pressure can help confirm the diagnosis. (Tonometry is omitted when there is an obvious external infection.)
9. Detect the presence of proptosis (Slide 35), lid malfunction, or any limitations of eye movement.

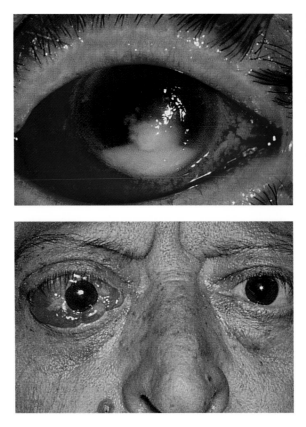

Slide 34   Corneal ulcer with hypopyon. This inflamed eye shows a white corneal opacity associated with an irregular corneal reflex. In addition, a prominent layering of purulent material appears in the inferior aspect of the anterior chamber, a hypopyon.

Slide 35   Chronic proptosis. The right eye of this patient is proptotic, or anteriorly displaced. Marked edema (chemosis) with hyperemia of the conjunctiva is also evident, with tissue prolapse over the lower lid margin. The patient has an orbital tumor.

How to Interpret the Findings

Although many conditions can cause a red eye, and the associated signs and symptoms of the various disorders overlap to some extent, several signs and symptoms signal danger. The presence of one or more of these danger signals should alert the physician that the patient has a disorder requiring an ophthalmologist's attention. Tables 4.1 and 4.2 summarize significant signs and symptoms in the differential diagnosis of a red eye. In the sections that follow, an exclamation point after a sign or symptom indicates a danger signal .

Signs of Red Eye

Reduced Visual Acuity ❶

Reduced visual acuity suggests a serious ocular disease, such as an inflamed cornea, iridocyclitis, or glaucoma. It never occurs in simple conjunctivitis unless there is associated corneal involvement.

Table 4.1 Signs of Red Eye

Sign	Referral Advisable if Present	Acute Glaucoma	Acute Iridocyclitis	Keratitis	Bacterial Conjunctivitis	Viral Conjunctivitis	Allergic Conjunctivitis
Ciliary flush	Yes	+	+	+	−	−	−
Conjunctival hyperemia	No	+	+	+	+	+	+
Corneal opacification	Yes	+	−	+	−	+/−	−
Corneal epithelial disruption	Yes	−	−	+	−	+/−	−
Pupillary abnormalities	Yes	+	+	+/−	−	−	−
Shallow anterior chamber depth	Yes	+	−	−	−	−	−
Elevated intraocular pressure	Yes	+	+/−	−	−	−	−
Proptosis	Yes	−	−	−	−	−	−
Discharge	No	−	−	+/−	+	+	+
Preauricular lymph-node enlargement	No	−	−	−	−	+	−

Note:
+ = Usually has sign
− = Does not usually have sign
+/− = May or may not have sign

Ciliary Flush ❽

Ciliary flush (see Slide 23) is an injection of the deep conjunctival and epi-scleral vessels surrounding the cornea. It is seen most easily in daylight and appears as a faint violaceous ring in which individual vessels are indiscernible to the unaided eye. Ciliary flush is a danger sign often seen in eyes with corneal inflammations, iridocyclitis, or acute glaucoma. Usually, ciliary flush is not present in conjunctivitis.

Conjunctival Hyperemia

Conjunctival hyperemia (see Slide 25) is an engorgement of the larger and more superficial bulbar conjunctival vessels. A nonspecific sign, it may be seen in almost any of the conditions causing a red eye.

Corneal Opacification ❽

In a patient with a red eye, corneal opacities always denote disease. These opacities may be detected by direct illumination with a penlight, or they may be seen with a direct ophthalmoscope (with a plus lens in the viewing aperture) outlined against the red fundus reflex. Several types of corneal opacities may occur:

Table 4.2   Symptoms of Red Eye

Symptom	Referral Advisable if Present	Acute Glaucoma	Acute Irido-cyclitis	Keratitis	Bacterial Conjunc-tivitis	Viral Conjunc-tivitis	Allergic Conjunc-tivitis
Blurred vision	Yes	3	1 to 2	3	0	0	0
Pain	Yes	2 to 3	2	2	0	0	0
Photophobia	Yes	1	3	3	0	0	0
Colored halos	Yes	2	0	0	0	0	0
Exudation	No	0	0	0 to 3	3	2	1
Itching	No	0	0	0	0	0	2 to 3

Note: The range of severity of the symptom is indicated by 0 (absent) to 3 (severe).

- Keratic precipitates, or cellular deposits on the corneal endothelium, usually too small to be visible but occasionally forming large clumps; these precipitates can result from iritis or from chronic iridocyclitis (see Slide 30)
- A diffuse haze obscuring the pupil and iris markings, characteristic of corneal edema (see Slide 31) and frequently seen in acute glaucoma
- Localized opacities due to keratitis or ulcer (see Slide 32)

Corneal Epithelial Disruption ❷

Disruption of the corneal epithelium occurs in corneal inflammations and trauma. It can be detected in two ways:

1. Position yourself so that you can observe the reflection from the cornea of a single light source (eg, window, penlight) as the patient moves the eye into various positions. Epithelial disruptions cause distortion and irregularity of the reflection (see Slide 33).
2. Apply fluorescein to the eye. Diseased epithelium or areas denuded of epithelium will stain a bright green. (See Slides 5 and 6 and accompanying text in Chapter 1 for the technique of fluorescein staining.)

Pupillary Abnormalities ❷

The pupil in an eye with iridocyclitis typically is somewhat smaller than that of the other eye, due to reflex spasm of the iris sphincter muscle. The pupil is also distorted occasionally by posterior synechiae, which are inflammatory adhesions between the lens and the iris. In acute glaucoma, the pupil is usually fixed, middilated (about 5 to 6 mm), and slightly irregular. Conjunctivitis does not affect the pupil.

Shallow Anterior Chamber Depth ❷

In a red eye, a shallow anterior chamber should always suggest the possibility of acute angle-closure glaucoma (see Slide 22). Anterior chamber depth can be estimated through side illumination with a penlight. If possible, compare the anterior chamber depth of the red eye with that of the other, unaffected eye. (See Chapter 1 for details on estimating the depth of the anterior chamber.)

Elevated Intraocular Pressure ✛

Intraocular pressure is unaffected by common causes of red eye other than iridocyclitis and glaucoma. Intraocular pressure should be measured when angle-closure glaucoma is suspected. (See Chapter 1 for the use of tonometry to measure intraocular pressure.)

Proptosis ✛

Proptosis is a forward displacement of the globe. Sudden proptosis suggests serious orbital or cavernous sinus disease; in children, orbital infection or tumor should be suspected. The most common cause of chronic proptosis is thyroid disease; however, orbital mass lesions also result in proptosis and should be ruled out early in the diagnosis (see Slide 35). Proptosis may be accompanied by conjunctival hyperemia or limitation of eye movement. Small amounts of proptosis are detected most easily by standing behind the seated patient and looking down to compare the positions of the two corneas.

Discharge

The type of discharge may be an important clue to the cause of a patient's conjunctivitis. Purulent (creamy-white, see Slide 29) or mucopurulent (yellowish) exudate suggests a bacterial cause. Serous (watery, clear or yellow-tinged) discharge suggests a viral cause. Scant, white, stringy discharge sometimes occurs in allergic conjunctivitis and in keratoconjunctivitis sicca, a condition commonly known as *dry eyes*.

Preauricular Lymph-Node Enlargement

Enlargement of the lymph node just in front of the auricle is a frequent sign of viral conjunctivitis. Usually, such enlargement does not occur in acute bacterial conjunctivitis. Preauricular node enlargement can be a prominent feature of some unusual varieties of chronic granulomatous conjunctivitis, known collectively as *Parinaud's oculoglandular syndrome*.

Symptoms of Red Eye

Blurred Vision ✛

Blurred vision often indicates serious ocular disease (see "Reduced Visual Acuity" in the preceding section, "Signs of Red Eye"). Blurred vision that improves with blinking suggests a discharge or mucus on the ocular surface.

Severe Pain ❷

Pain may indicate keratitis, ulcer, iridocyclitis, or acute glaucoma. Patients with conjunctivitis may complain of a scratchiness or mild irritation but not of severe pain.

Photophobia ❷

Photophobia is an abnormal sensitivity to light that accompanies iritis, either alone or secondary to corneal inflammation. Patients with conjunctivitis have normal light sensitivity.

Colored Halos ❷

Rainbow-like fringes or colored halos seen around a point of light are usually a symptom of corneal edema, often resulting from an abrupt rise in intraocular pressure. Therefore, colored halos are a danger symptom suggesting acute glaucoma as the cause of a red eye.

Exudation

Exudation, also called *mattering*, is a typical result of conjunctival or eyelid inflammation and does not occur in iridocyclitis or glaucoma. Patients will often complain that their lids are "stuck together" on awakening from sleep. Corneal ulcer is a serious condition that may or may not be accompanied by exudate.

Itching

Although it is a nonspecific symptom, itching usually indicates an allergic conjunctivitis.

Associated Systemic Problems

Upper Respiratory Tract Infection and Fever

Infection of the upper respiratory tract accompanied by fever may be associated with conjunctivitis, particularly when these symptoms are due to adenovirus type 3 or type 7 (both of which cause pharyngoconjunctival fever). Allergic conjunctivitis may be associated with the seasonal rhinitis of hay fever.

Erythema Multiforme

Erythema multiforme is a serious systemic disorder, possibly an allergic response to medication, which can result in severe conjunctivitis, irreversible conjunctival scarring, and blindness. In erythema multiforme, bull's-eye or target-shaped red lesions are found on the skin. The name *Stevens-Johnson syndrome* is given to the form of erythema multiforme associated with ocular involvement.

Laboratory Diagnosis

In practice, most mild cases of conjunctivitis are managed without laboratory assistance. This represents a compromise with ideal management but is justified by the economic waste of obtaining routine smears and cultures in such a common and benign disease. Most clinicians, after making a presumptive clinical diagnosis of bacterial conjunctivitis, proceed directly to broad-spectrum topical ophthalmic antibiotic treatment. Cases of presumed bacterial conjunctivitis that do not improve after 2 days of antibiotic treatment should be referred to an ophthalmologist for confirmation of the diagnosis and appropriate laboratory studies. In addition, in cases of hyperpurulent conjunctivitis, when copious purulent discharge is produced, conjunctival cultures and ophthalmologic consultation are indicated because of a possible gonococcal cause. Gonococcal hyperpurulent conjunctivitis is a serious, potentially blinding disease.

In doubtful cases, smears of exudate or conjunctival scrapings can confirm clinical impressions regarding the type of conjunctivitis. Typical findings include polymorphonuclear cells and bacteria in bacterial conjunctivitis, lymphocytes in viral conjunctivitis, and eosinophils in allergic conjunctivitis. Cultures for bacteria and determinations of antibiotic sensitivity are also useful in cases resistant to therapy.

Management or Referral

The following conditions either require no treatment or may be appropriately treated by a primary care physician. Patients with chronic, unilateral blepharitis should be referred to an ophthalmologist to rule out a malignant process such as sebaceous cell carcinoma or squamous cell carcinoma. Cases requiring prolonged treatment or those in which the expected response to treatment does not occur promptly should also be referred to an ophthalmologist.

Blepharitis

Response to the treatment of blepharitis, or inflammation of the eyelid, is often frustratingly slow, and relapses are common. The mainstays of treatment are

- Eradication of staphylococcal infection (Slide 36) with frequent applications of appropriate antibiotic eyedrops or ointment
- Treatment of scalp seborrhea with antidandruff shampoos to prevent the spread of seborrhea to the eyes
- Cleansing of the lids to alleviate seborrheic blepharitis (Slide 37)

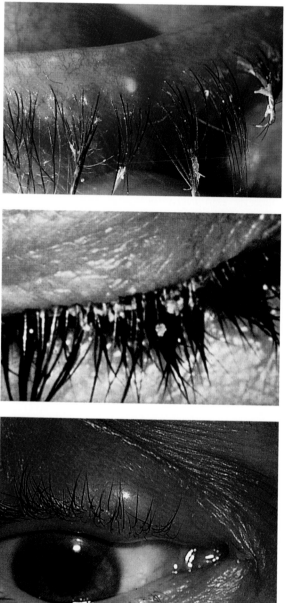

Slide 36 Staphylococcal blepharitis. Chronic staphylococcal lid infection produces inflamed, swollen lids that may ulcerate. The oily discharge binds the lashes and sometimes condenses to form a collarette around a lash.

Slide 37 Seborrheic blepharitis. The dry, flaky lashes and red lid margins seen here are characteristic of seborrheic blepharitis.

Slide 38 External hordeolum. This large, acute swelling, which is red and painful, involves the hair follicles or associated glands of Zeis or Moll and points toward the skin.

Stye and Chalazion

A stye, or hordeolum, is an acute inflammation of the glands or hair follicles in the eyelid. Hordeola can be categorized as external or internal according to where the inflammation is located in the lid (Slides 38 and 39). A chalazion is a chronic inflammation of a meibomian gland in the eyelid that may develop spontaneously or may follow a hordeolum (Slide 40).

Styes are initially treated with hot compresses. Topical antibiotics can be used if the lesion is tender and infection is suspected. However, most styes

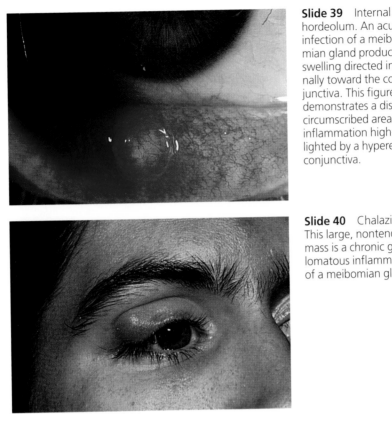

Slide 39 Internal hordeolum. An acute infection of a meibomian gland produces a swelling directed internally toward the conjunctiva. This figure demonstrates a discrete, circumscribed area of inflammation highlighted by a hyperemic conjunctiva.

Slide 40 Chalazion. This large, nontender lid mass is a chronic granulomatous inflammation of a meibomian gland.

and chalazia are sterile inflammatory reactions. Incision with curettage is indicated when lesions do not resolve spontaneously or with medical therapy. A persistent or recurring lid mass should undergo biopsy because it may be a rare meibomian gland carcinoma or squamous cell carcinoma of the lid rather than a benign chalazion.

Subconjunctival Hemorrhage

In the absence of blunt trauma, hemorrhage into the subconjunctiva, the potential space between the conjunctiva and the sclera, requires no treatment and, unless recurrent, no evaluation. (See Slide 49 in Chapter 5.) Causes include a sudden increase in ocular venous pressure, such as occurs with coughing, sneezing, vomiting, or vigorous rubbing of the eye. Many subconjunctival hemorrhages occur during sleep. If recurrent, an underlying bleeding disorder should be considered.

Conjunctivitis

Bacterial conjunctivitis is treated with frequent antibiotic eyedrops as well as antibiotic ointment applied at bedtime. Cool compresses may give some relief. There is no specific medicinal treatment for viral conjunctivitis, although patients should be instructed in proper precautions to prevent contagion. It cannot be emphasized too strongly that corticosteroids have no place in the treatment of infectious conjunctivitis and that eyedrops containing a combination of antibiotics and corticosteroids are seldom indicated for the treatment of ocular inflammation.

Therapeutic Warnings

Topical Anesthetics

Topical anesthetics should *never* be prescribed for prolonged analgesia in ocular inflammations and injuries for three reasons:

1. Topical anesthetics inhibit growth and healing of the corneal epithelium.
2. Although rare, severe allergic reaction may result from instillation of topical anesthetics.
3. Corneal anesthesia eliminates the protective blink reflex, exposing the cornea to dehydration, injury, and infection.

Topical Corticosteroids

Topical corticosteroids have three potentially serious ocular side effects:

1. **Keratitis**   Both herpes simplex keratitis (see Slide 24) and fungal keratitis are markedly potentiated by corticosteroids. Corticosteroids may mask symptoms of inflammation, making the patient "feel" better, while the cornea may be melting away or even perforating.
2. **Cataract**   Prolonged use of corticosteroids, either locally or systemically, will often lead to cataract formation.
3. **Elevated intraocular pressure**   Local application of corticosteroids for 2 to 6 weeks may cause an elevation of intraocular pressure in approximately one third of the population. The pressure rise may be severe in a small percentage of cases. Optic nerve damage and permanent loss of vision can occur.

The combination of a corticosteroid and an antibiotic carries the same risk. Topical corticosteroids alone or in combination with antibiotics should not be administered to the eye by a primary care physician. They can be very helpful when used under the close supervision of an ophthalmologist.

Points to Remember

1. If visual acuity is acutely and significantly reduced, a diagnosis of conjunctivitis is extremely unlikely.
2. Fluorescein should always be instilled in a red eye to test for integrity of the corneal epithelium.
3. A pupillary inequality in a patient with red eye(s) is a danger signal for serious ocular disease.

Sample Problems

1. A 23-year-old school teacher complains that her right eye is red and irritated. You note moderate injection of the larger conjunctival vessels, watery discharge, and a palpable preauricular lymph node.

   A. From this information alone, what tentative diagnosis would you make?

   Answer: The conjunctival injection and discharge suggest conjunctivitis. The serous nature of the discharge plus the preauricular adenopathy indicate that she has viral conjunctivitis.

   B. Again based on the above information, which of the following symptoms or facts might be elicited by careful history-taking?
      a. Blurred vision
      b. Sore throat
      c. Exposure to children with colds
      d. Itching

   Answer: b and c. Sore throat often accompanies viral conjunctivitis; in such cases, a history of exposure to other individuals with upper respiratory tract infections can often be elicited. Blurred vision, a danger signal of serious ocular disease, is not a feature of simple conjunctivitis. Itching is a symptom of allergic, not viral, conjunctivitis.

   C. Which of the following are also likely findings in this case of viral conjunctivitis?
      a. A small pupil in the right eye
      b. Lymphocytes in a smear of conjunctival scrapings
      c. Keratic precipitates

   Answer: b. Lymphocytes are usually found in scrapings from eyes with viral conjunctivitis. A small pupil and keratic precipitates are signs of iritis.

   D. Management by a primary care physician should consist of which of the following?
      a. Corticosteroid eyedrops
      b. Broad-spectrum antibiotic eyedrops
      c. Referral to an ophthalmologist
      d. Instruction to the patient to use cool compresses and stay home from school until the redness resolves

   Answer: d. Because the disease is contagious, the patient should be instructed to remain home from work. There is no specific medicinal treatment for viral conjunctivitis. Corticosteroids are contraindicated.

2. A man returned recently from an African journey. During his trip he had three episodes of blurring and pain in his left eye; each episode lasted about 2 hours and was relieved by sleep. A few hours before consulting you, his symptoms recurred.

A. Which of the following signs convince you that the patient does not have conjunctivitis?
   a. Visual acuity of 20/200 in the left eye
   b. Conjunctival injection
   c. Ciliary flush
   d. Absence of exudate

Answer: a and c. Reduced visual acuity, as well as ciliary flush, often signals ocular disease more serious than conjunctivitis.

B. You note a diffuse haziness of the patient's left cornea. What is the most likely diagnosis?

Answer: Diffuse haziness of the cornea is usually due to edema. This and the history of recurrent attacks relieved by sleep suggest the diagnosis of acute angle-closure glaucoma.

C. You seek confirmatory data for your tentative diagnosis. What do you expect the following tests to show if your diagnosis is correct?
   a. Estimation of anterior chamber depth: deep or shallow?
   b. Determination of pupil diameter: large, middilated, or small?
   c. Measurement of intraocular pressure: high or low?

Answer: In angle-closure glaucoma, the anterior chamber is *shallow,* the pupil is usually *middilated,* and the intraocular pressure is *high.*

D. Your management should be which of the following?
   a. Corticosteroid eyedrops
   b. Advice to see an ophthalmologist the next day
   c. A telephone request to an ophthalmologist for immediate examination

Answer: c. Angle-closure glaucoma requires emergency treatment to lower the intraocular pressure. The patient should be referred immediately to an ophthalmologist. If an ophthalmologist is not immediately available, you may begin topical pilocarpine hydrochloride 1% or 2%, a topical beta-adrenergic blocker, and a systemic carbonic anhydrase inhibitor. (See Chapter 9 for details on these drugs.)

3. After working in his garden, a 57-year-old man complains of moderate discomfort and redness in his right eye. You note a visual acuity of 20/25 in the right eye and 20/15 in the left eye. The right eye has mild hyperemia of the conjunctival vessels; the right cornea appears clear to penlight examination. You diagnose a probable allergy to pollen and advise the patient to use topical dexamethasone sodium phosphate 0.1% for 3 days.

A. Give two reasons why your diagnosis of allergic conjunctivitis is unlikely to be correct.

Answer: Unless the patient has always had weaker vision in his right eye, this finding should alert you to the possibility of a more serious inflammation, such as iritis, keratitis, or glaucoma. Also, the patient did not complain of itching, which you might expect in an allergic reaction.

B. What other diagnostic techniques should you have performed to be certain that the cornea is normal?

Answer: If the patient has an early herpes simplex keratitis or if his cornea has been scratched by a twig, the epithelial disruption might not be easily seen during a penlight examination. However, it most likely would be rendered visible by fluorescein staining of the cornea.

C. Is there any hazard in your prescribed course of treatment? Explain.

Answer: Yes. The virulence of both herpes simplex and fungal infections, which can result from trauma involving organic material, is markedly potentiated by the application of topical corticosteroids to the eye.

4. A 38-year-old woman complains of a 3-day history of a red, tender right eyelid. Physical examination reveals a tender nodule of the right lower eyelid with minimal injection of the inferior conjunctiva.
   A. Which of the following would constitute appropriate management by the primary care physician? (More than one course of action may be possible.)
   a. hot compresses
   b. broad-spectrum systemic antibiotics
   c. topical antibiotics
   d. immediate surgical incision and drainage to prevent cellulitis

   Answer: a and c. The patient has a stye. Because she has only had symptoms for 3 days and the lesion is tender to touch, she would benefit from hot compresses. Topical antibiotic ointment might benefit a small percentage of patients. Incision and drainage is indicated only when lesions do not resolve spontaneously or with medical therapy. Usually surgical intervention occurs only after the lesion has been present for several weeks. Systemic antibiotics are not indicated.

   B. If the patient reports she has had numerous nodules in this same area over the last 5 years, how should the primary care physician change the management plan?

   Answer: A persistent or recurring lid mass should undergo biopsy to rule out an eyelid malignancy. Referral to an ophthalmologist is indicated.

Annotated Resources

Albert DM, Jakobiec FA, eds: *Principles and Practice of Ophthalmology.* Philadelphia: WB Saunders Co; 1993. Chapters with information relevant to red eye conditions include Chapter 6, "Viral Disease of the Cornea and External Eye"; Chapter 7, "Bacterial Infections of the Conjunctiva and Cornea"; and Chapter 152, "Eyelid Infections."

Newell FW: *Ophthalmology: Principles and Concepts.* 8th ed. St Louis: CV Mosby Co; 1996. This comprehensive text includes detailed discussions of diseases of the conjunctiva and cornea.

Tasman W, Jaeger EA, eds: *Duane's Clinical Ophthalmology*. Philadelphia: JB Lippincott Co; 1991, vol 4. Updated, comprehensive discussions of various forms of conjunctivitis are found in Chapters 4 to 9A and of anterior uveitis in Chapters 39 to 42.

Trobe JD: *The Physician's Guide to Eye Care*. San Francisco: American Academy of Ophthalmology; 1993. A brief but comprehensive resource covering the principal clinical ophthalmic problems that nonophthalmologist physicians are likely to encounter, organized for practical use by practitioners.

Chapter 5

Ocular and Orbital Injuries

Objectives

As a primary care physician, you should be able to evaluate the common ocular or orbital injuries and to determine whether or not the problem requires the prompt attention of an ophthalmologist. In situations of true ocular emergency, such as chemical burns, you should be able to institute therapy when necessary.

To achieve these objectives, you should learn

- To recognize which problems are emergent or urgent and deal with them accordingly
- To obtain the salient historical facts
- How to examine the traumatized eye
- To record the visual acuity as accurately as possible
- How to determine whether to manage or to refer the most common injuries

Relevance

One day, whether in your own home or yard or while on duty in the emergency center, you will be confronted with an unexpected ocular injury. Your skill in dealing with major eye injuries can mean the difference between preservation and loss of a patient's vision. The purpose of this chapter is to assist in developing confidence when approaching minor or major eye injuries; it will further your competence in acquiring the basic techniques and knowledge necessary to assess and initiate treatment of the eye and its surrounding structures.

Basic Information

Anatomy and Function

Bony Orbit

- The orbit is the bony, concave cavity in the skull that houses the globe, the extraocular muscles, and the blood vessels and nerves of the eye (Figure 5.1).
- The rim of the orbit protects the globe from impact with large objects.

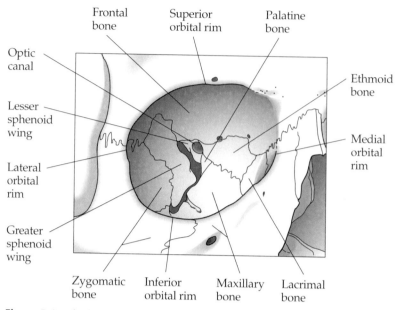

Figure 5.1   The bony orbit.

- A rim fracture usually causes no decrease in ocular or visual function.
- The very thin orbital floor (consisting of the maxillary, palatine, and zygomatic bones) may "blow out" into the maxillary sinus from blunt impact to the orbit, for instance, from a fist or tennis ball. Orbital contents, including the inferior rectus and inferior oblique muscles, may become trapped, restricting vertical eye movement and causing double vision (diplopia).
- A medial fracture of the thin ethmoidal bone may be associated with subcutaneous emphysema of the eyelids.
- A fracture at or near the optic canal, through which the optic nerve and ophthalmic artery pass, may cause damage to the optic nerve or the vessels that supply it (traumatic optic neuropathy), with resulting visual loss.

Eyelids

- The lids close reflexively when the eyes are threatened.
- The act of blinking keeps the cornea clear through constant surface contact and tear production.
- In the case of a facial nerve palsy, the globe may be exposed to drying or other injury.
- Lid margins must be intact to ensure proper lid closure and tear drainage.

Lacrimal Apparatus

- Tear drainage occurs at the medial aspect of the lids, primarily through the lower lacrimal punctum, and continues through the canaliculi to the lacrimal sac, and via the nasolacrimal duct to the nose (see Figure 1.2 in Chapter 1).
- Failure to recognize and properly repair a canalicular laceration can result in chronic tearing (epiphora).

Conjunctiva and Cornea

- The corneal epithelium usually heals quickly following abrasion.
- Small lacerations of the conjunctiva heal quickly and, consequently, may conceal a penetrating injury of the globe.

Anterior Chamber

- The aqueous humor often escapes in penetrating injuries, sometimes resulting in a shallow or flat chamber.

Iris and Ciliary Body

- Following laceration of the cornea or limbus, the iris may prolapse into the wound (Slide 41), resulting in an irregular pupil.
- Blunt trauma to the eyeball may produce iritis, resulting in pain, redness, photophobia, and a small pupil (miosis).
- Contusions may deform the pupil by tearing the iris root or by notching the pupillary margin.
- Contusions may result in tearing of small vessels in the anterior chamber angle, causing hemorrhage into the anterior chamber (hyphema, Slide 42). A hyphema is generally the result of trauma and usually resolves spontaneously.

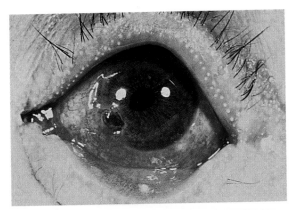

Slide 41 Corneal perforation with iris prolapse. Slight distortion of the pupil, irregularity of the corneal reflection, and a knuckle of soft, brown tissue at the limbus indicate a corneal perforation through which the iris has prolapsed.

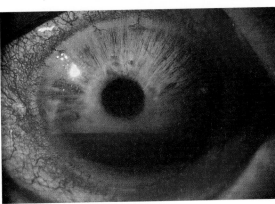

Slide 42 Hyphema. In the anterior chamber at the 6-o'clock position, a dark pool of blood with a flat top is visible. Note also the conjunctival hyperemia.

Lens

- Injuries to the lens usually proceed to cataract formation.
- Blunt trauma to the globe can cause a partial dislocation (subluxation) of the lens (Slide 43).

Vitreous Humor

- Loss of transparency may be observed in the presence of hemorrhage, inflammation, or infection.

Retina

- The retina is protected externally by the sclera (a tough outer layer) and the choroid (an underlying vascular layer).
- The retina is thin and vulnerable. If the surface is scratched or has been penetrated by a foreign body, retinal detachment may occur (see discussion and Slide 7 in Chapter 2).
- Retinal hemorrhage may develop as a result of direct or indirect trauma.
- The retina turns white when edematous.
- Macular damage will reduce visual acuity without producing complete blindness.

When to Examine

Most ocular injuries present with obvious redness and pain. However, not all injuries provide such obvious warning signs. For example, a sharp perforation may produce minimal redness and escape attention. The examiner should be especially alert to perforating injuries caused by small projectiles resulting from metal striking metal. An intraocular foreign body (Slide 44) produces no pain because the lens, retina, and vitreous have no nerve endings to conduct sensations of pain.

If disease of the posterior segment is suspected, including retinal detachment or intraocular foreign body, referral to an ophthalmologist is

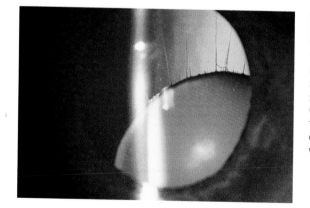

Slide 43 Subluxated lens. Light reflected off the fundus and back through a dilated pupil silhouettes the edge of a subluxated lens with stretched zonular fibers. Ordinarily, the edge of the lens is not visible even if the pupil is widely dilated.

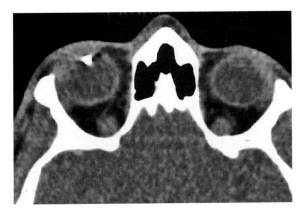

Slide 44   CT scan of foreign body. A small, radiopaque intraocular foreign body is visible in the anterior segment of the eye.

indicated. The ophthalmologist's examination of the fundus will be facilitated if you do not use ointment in the eye.

How to Examine

For an eye injury, you should obtain a patient history if possible, and perform a complete examination of the eyes and surrounding structures. This should include visual acuity, external examination, the pupils, eye movements, and ophthalmoscopy. Two sample examinations are provided in Tables 5.1 and 5.2.

History

In the evaluation of ocular injuries, it is important to document the type of traumatic event as well as the time of onset and the nature of the symptoms. Specific historical information to obtain includes the time, place, and type of injury (eg, blunt or sharp trauma; acid or alkali burn) and the patient's history of eye conditions, drug allergies, and tetanus immunization. As in any trauma situation, you should not delay prompt treatment for a detailed history if an obvious injury, such as a chemical burn, exists.

After significant trauma has occurred, the patient may be unconscious or unable to answer questions. In this case, the physician can question whoever accompanied the patient for as much historical information as possible, but must be prepared to assess the injury and proceed with treatment or referral in the absence of adequate historical information.

Visual Acuity Testing

Visual acuity should be recorded as specifically as possible. Refer to Chapter 1 for instructions on the use of the Snellen eye chart. If a Snellen chart is unavailable, determine the patient's ability to read available print material and record the type of print used (eg, newspaper, telephone book) and the

Table 5.1 *Sample Examination: Foreign-Body Sensation*

History

Type of injury, time, and place	Foreign-body sensation, 3:15 AM, seen in emergency center
Pertinent chain of events Is trauma centered in OD, OS, or OU?	At about 2:45 AM, patient awoke with severe foreign-body sensation OU
Subjective visual loss, if any, and amount of visual decrease Associated complaints, symptoms	No injury, although admits to using sunlamp to tan face for 20 minutes previous evening. Now unable to open eyes, which aggravates burning foreign-body sensation. Unable to see well but uncertain about
Was vision normal prior to injury?	degree of visual loss. Patient states vision has been normal until now.

Examination

Best correctable VA for both eyes, ie, with glasses if available, with pinhole if necessary	Unable to cooperate until 1 drop proparacaine 0.5% administered OU VA: OD 20/25; OS 20/20
Appearance and function of:	
Bony orbit and lids	Bony orbit intact Marked eyelid spasm until anesthetic drops given
Cornea and conjunctiva	Cornea stains irregularly with fluorescein Conjunctival injection OU, pronounced near limbus
Media (aqueous, lens, vitreous)	Media clear on gross inspection

Diagnosis	Ultraviolet conjunctival and corneal injury

Management	Cycloplegic drops, antibiotic ointment, and moderate pressure dressing

distance at which it was read. Note in particular whether vision is equal in both eyes. If vision is below reading level, determine the patient's ability to count fingers, perceive hand motions, or respond to light.

External Examination

An examination of the external structures of the eye may include palpation, penlight inspection, lid eversion, fluorescein staining, and topical anesthesia. Palpation of the orbital rims should be performed if a blunt injury or fracture is suspected. A penlight is used to inspect the eye for signs of perforation, such as reduced depth of the anterior chamber or uveal prolapse (see Slide 41). Hyphema (see Slide 42) may be present without perforation and, in fact, often accompanies blunt injury. Lid eversion (retraction and eversion of the upper and lower eyelids) will facilitate

Table 5.2 Sample Examination: Double Vision

History	
Approximate onset of symptoms	A 16-year-old boy complains that he awoke 2 days ago with fullness OS. Later, he noted vertical double vision when looking straight up, up and right, and up and left; no double vision when looking straight ahead. No other problem except mild aching when looking up. Hit by knee in left eye in wrestling class 3 days earlier. Symptoms unchanged since first noted.
Type of symptoms, frequency, regularity	
Increasing or decreasing severity?	

Examination	
Ocular findings	Perform complete eye examination, with particular attention to testing extraocular muscles. Rule out possible damage to the globe. Patient unable to elevate left eye beyond primary gaze. Globe examination unremarkable except for localized subconjunctival hemorrhage. Visual acuity normal.
X-rays	Obtain Waters view, which reveals opacification of the maxillary antrum and downward herniation of orbital structures. CT scan more clearly delineates fracture of orbital floor.

Diagnosis	Blowout fracture left orbit with muscle entrapment.

Management	Call ophthalmologist. Patient should be evaluated semiurgently for consideration of surgical repair.

inspection for a foreign body or chemical burn. *Do not manipulate the eyelids if you suspect a penetrating injury of the globe.*

If the patient has a foreign-body sensation or if there is a history of blunt or sharp injury, fluorescein is used to stain the cornea to identify any corneal epithelial defects. (See Chapter 1 for the technique of fluorescein staining.)

Drops can be used to provide topical anesthesia, especially to relieve foreign-body sensation or discomfort due to radiant energy burns or prolonged wear of contact lenses. Use of 1 drop of proparacaine hydrochloride 0.5% will provide almost instantaneous pain relief and allow you to proceed with an adequate evaluation, including determination of visual acuity, which would otherwise be impossible due to discomfort. Do not prescribe or distribute samples of anesthetic drops or ointment because prolonged use can result in corneal ulceration and inadvertent injury.

Pupillary Reactions

Always check pupillary reactions in trauma cases. Diminished direct pupillary reaction to light with an intact consensual response (a relative afferent pupillary defect) may indicate an optic nerve injury (see Chapter 7).

Ocular Motility Testing

Movement of the eye may be generally restricted in the case of orbital hematoma. Vertical restriction combined with vertical diplopia should make you suspect a blowout fracture. If limitation of eye movements is accompanied by proptosis, auscultate the head and eye for a bruit, which would be suggestive of a carotid–cavernous sinus fistula.

Ophthalmoscopy

If the fundus is visible, look for edema, retinal hemorrhages, retinal detachment, and, if penetration is suspected, a foreign body. In the event of a positive finding or the suspicion of a penetrating injury or foreign body, refer the patient to an ophthalmologist immediately.

The normal red reflex from the fundus is evenly colored and not interrupted by shadows (see Slide 1 in Chapter 1). If the red reflex is absent, immediate referral to an ophthalmologist is indicated. Absence of the red reflex may be due to hyphema in the anterior chamber, cataract from acute swelling of the lens, or vitreous hemorrhage. Hyphema is visible on external examination with a penlight, whereas the detection of cataract and vitreous hemorrhage requires assessment with a direct ophthalmoscope.

Pupillary dilation to permit evaluation of the fundus should be routine. The only general exceptions to this rule would be in patients with head trauma where pupillary signs might be important for neurologic evaluation and patients whose shallow anterior chamber predisposes them for narrow-angle glaucoma.

Radiologic Studies

Radiologic evaluation is suggested if there is any question of facial or orbital fracture or of ocular or orbital foreign body. A CT scan can often provide additional useful detail. MRI should not be ordered if a metallic foreign body is suspected, because the metal may heat, vibrate, or move during the scan, resulting in additional intraocular injury.

Management or Referral

The primary care physician may not be able to provide definitive care for each of the entities discussed below, but should be able to initiate treatment in every case.

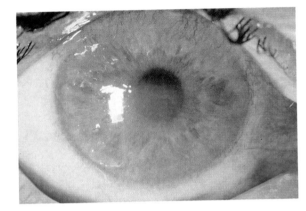

Slide 45   Alkali burn. Blanching of the conjunctiva and a large corneal epithelial defect, demonstrated by application of fluorescein, indicate a relatively serious injury.

True Emergency

Therapy must be instituted within minutes. A chemical burn of the conjunctiva and cornea represents one of the true ocular emergencies. An alkali burn (Slide 45) usually results in greater damage to the eye than an acid burn, because alkali compounds (eg, lye, anhydrous ammonia) penetrate ocular tissues more rapidly. All chemical burns require immediate and profuse irrigation, followed by referral to an ophthalmologist.

Urgent Situation

Urgent situations require therapy to be instituted within a few hours. The following list describes common urgent ocular situations and appropriate actions to take for each.

- Penetrating injuries of the globe, whether actual or suspected, necessitate the protection of an eye shield. Neither a patch nor an ointment is advisable. An x-ray or CT scan of the orbit to check for radiopaque foreign bodies (see Slide 44) should be ordered. Referral to an ophthalmologist is indicated.
- Conjunctival or corneal foreign bodies (Slides 46 and 47) require topical anesthetization followed by removal of the object with either vigorous irrigation or a cotton-tipped applicator. See "Foreign-Body Removal," below, for specific instructions.
- For corneal abrasions, take the following steps:
  1. Anesthetize with proparacaine 0.5%.
  2. Perform a gross examination.
  3. Stain with fluorescein to enhance the view. (For a depiction of a fluorescein stain delineating a corneal abrasion, see Slides 5 and 6 in Chapter 1.)
  4. Instill antibiotic drops; instill short-acting cycloplegic drops for the relief of pain as indicated.
  5. Some physicians apply a pressure patch to maintain lid closure for 24 hours, although others feel that abrasions less than 10 mm in diameter heal better and more quickly without a pressure patch.
  6. Refer severe cases to an ophthalmologist.
- Hyphema requires immediate referral to an ophthalmologist. Elevation of intraocular pressure may necessitate medical or surgical intervention.

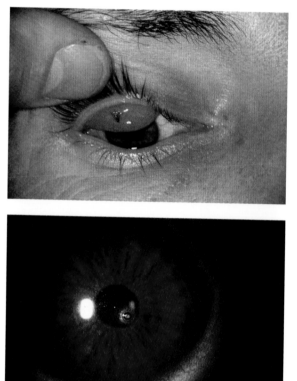

Slide 46 Conjunctival foreign body. A foreign body often lodges under the edge of the upper eyelid. As this figure shows, the foreign body is easily seen and removed upon eversion of the eyelid.

Slide 47 Corneal foreign body. Visible here is a small piece of iron embedded in the surface of the cornea. Surrounding the iron are a ring of rust and grayish corneal edema.

Also, the hyphema may be a sign of globe rupture or some other, initially obscure, serious ocular injuries, such as dislocated lens or retinal detachment.

- A lid laceration can be sutured if not deep and neither the lid margin nor the canaliculi are involved; otherwise, refer to an ophthalmologist. (The lid laceration shown in Slide 48 would require referral because it is full-thickness and involves the lid margin. There is also a possibility of canalicular involvement because the laceration is close to the medial canthus.)
- Radiant energy burns, such as welder's burn or snow blindness, require topical anesthesia, examination, topical antibiotic and cycloplegic agents, and patching. (See Chapter 9 for information about instilling ocular medications.)
- Traumatic optic neuropathy, although uncommon, should always be considered in patients with cranial or maxillofacial trauma. Patients present with a history of facial or frontal trauma, usually with unilateral decreased vision and a relative afferent pupillary defect, but further examination reveals no clear ocular origin. High-resolution CT imaging of the orbital apex, optic canal, and cavernous sinus is essential if traumatic optic neuropathy is suspected. Patients may benefit from intravenous high-dose methylprednisolone if given in the first 8 hours after initial injury. If a patient is suspected of having traumatic optic neuropathy, a prompt referral to an ophthalmologist is indicated.

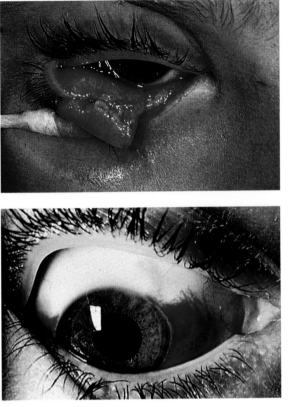

Slide 48 Full-thickness lid laceration. The lower eyelid is partially everted with the applicator stick, revealing an irregular laceration of the lid margin, orbicularis muscle, tarsal plate, and conjunctiva. Note the proximity of the laceration to the medial canthus, indicating possible canalicular involvement.

Slide 49 Subconjunctival hemorrhage. This circumscribed hemorrhage is located between the conjunctiva and the sclera; the history of a sudden appearance and the bright red color are characteristic.

Semiurgent Condition

Refer patients with semiurgent conditions to an ophthalmologist within 1 to 2 days. An orbital fracture falls in this category. Subconjunctival hemorrhage (Slide 49) in the presence of blunt trauma is also a semiurgent condition, unless a globe rupture or intraocular hemorrhage is suspected, in which case urgent referral to an ophthalmologist is indicated.

Treatment Skills

To manage eye injuries properly, every physician should be proficient in ocular irrigation, foreign-body removal, eye medication prescription, patching, and suturing.

Ocular Irrigation

Plastic squeeze bottles (Slide 50) of eye irrigation solutions and normal saline IV drip with plastic tubing are ideal for ocular irrigation. Irrigation may be facilitated by the use of a topical anesthetic. However, first aid for chemical injuries of the eye may demand the earliest possible irrigation using any source of water available, such as a garden hose, drinking

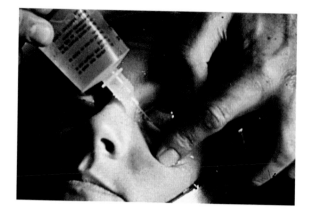

Slide 50 Irrigation. Here the examiner uses a plastic squeeze bottle of water or normal saline to irrigate the eye. The patient is instructed to look in various directions while the opposite portions of the conjunctival cul-de-sac are flushed vigorously.

fountain, or faucet. It cannot be overstated that chemical burns require immediate and profuse irrigation. Always direct the irrigating stream toward the temple and away from an unaffected fellow eye.

Foreign-Body Removal

To remove a superficial foreign body from the cornea or conjunctiva, instill an anesthetic such as proparacaine 0.5% and then gently roll a cotton-tipped applicator across the globe to pick up the object. A forceful stream of irrigating solution delivered from a squeeze bottle will often dislodge a superficial conjunctival or corneal foreign body. A sharper instrument may be required if the foreign body remains embedded, and referral to an ophthalmologist should be considered. The orange-brown "rust ring" resulting from an embedded iron foreign body is a common problem that requires special attention.

Eye Medication Prescription

All physicians should be able to prescribe or administer confidently the following ocular drugs. (See Chapter 9 for more detailed discussions and for the method of administering topical ocular drugs.)

- **Cycloplegics**   Homatropine hydrobromide 2% or cyclopentolate hydrochloride 1% may be used to relax the iris and ciliary body and to relieve the pain and discomfort of most forms of nonpenetrating ocular injuries. Longer-acting cycloplegics (eg, atropine) are usually contraindicated.
- **Antibiotic ointment**   In general, if employed for one-time use in clean wounds, antibiotic ointments can be used safely without side effects. If more frequent use is necessary, the possibility of allergic reactions or superinfections must be considered.
- **Anesthetic drops and ointment**   Ocular anesthetics should never be prescribed for home use because they are toxic to the corneal epithelium when used repeatedly.

Patching

- **Pressure patch** A moderate pressure patch is used following injuries that affect the corneal epithelium (eg, corneal abrasions) and after removal of foreign bodies. Two eye patches or one eye patch plus a fluffed piece of gauze is applied by putting moderate tension on the strips of tape used (Slide 51). Make sure the patch is tight enough to prevent the patient from inadvertently opening the eye under it. The patch should not be so tight as to cause the patient discomfort or severely compress the globe, which can compromise the retinal blood flow.
- **Shield** For more serious ocular injuries, such as penetration of the globe or hyphema, a shield should be taped over the eye as an interim measure to protect the eye from rubbing, pressure, and further injury prior to treatment by an ophthalmologist. The shield may consist of a perforated, malleable piece of metal (Slide 52), plastic, or a trimmed-down paper cup.

Suturing

Suturing of any eyelid skin laceration that does not involve the eyelid margin or the lacrimal canaliculi can be performed by the primary care physician. More complicated lid lacerations should be referred to an ophthalmologist.

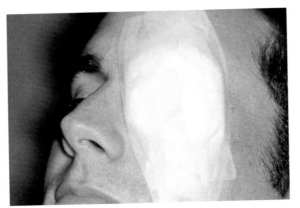

Slide 51 Pressure patch. The patient is instructed to close the affected eye while one or more oval, gauze eye patches are taped firmly enough to immobilize the lid in a closed position.

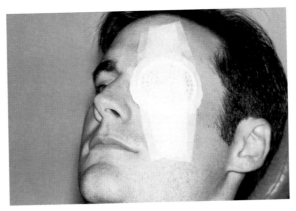

Slide 52 Shield. Shown here is the Fox shield, made of malleable metal and perforated. The shield is carefully shaped so that it is supported by the rim of the orbit when taped in place.

Points to Remember

1. Know your limits: Do not attempt complex repair, and know the results of inadequate repair.
2. Almost without fail, a teardrop-shaped pupil and a flat anterior chamber in an injured eye are associated with a perforating injury of the cornea or of the limbal area. Look for prolapse of dark tissue (either iris or ciliary body) at the point of the teardrop.
3. Avoid digital palpation of the globe in the patient who may have a corneal laceration or other perforating injury.
4. In a patient with a chemical burn, immediate irrigation is crucial just as soon as the nature of the injury has been learned. Do not attempt to neutralize or buffer the chemical substance. The goal is simply to dilute the chemical as thoroughly as possible by copious flushing.

Sample Problems

1. Your neighbor, a 43-year-old woman, is cleaning her swimming pool. While pouring some concentrated algicide into the pool, a large dollop of this solution splashes into her right eye. You are mowing your lawn when you hear her screams. You come to her aid less than 30 seconds after the injury. Which of the following should you do first?
   a. Bundle her into your car and speed off for the nearest emergency center.
   b. Run back home to get your medical bag where you keep a squeeze bottle of ophthalmic irrigating solution that you can use to flush out her eye.
   c. Run back to your study to look up the specific antidote for algicide.
   d. Carefully examine her eye for evidence of ocular hyperemia.
   e. Dunk her head into the swimming pool, instructing her to hold her eyes open to flush out the chemical.

   Answer: e. This is one of the few true emergencies of all the ocular injuries that you must know. Early and copious irrigation with whatever source of water is handy is the right approach to this problem. Even with prompt treatment, serious ocular injuries and visual damage may result, depending on the offending chemical. Time is of the essence. Do not resort to methods that will cause delay.

2. You are on duty in the emergency center when an 18-year-old high school student comes in because of pain, tearing, sensitivity to light, and blurred vision in his right eye. His symptoms began sometime that afternoon. Earlier, he had been working on his car and he remembers something flying into his right eye while he was trying to knock a rivet off the chassis with a hammer and chisel. You examine his eye and take visual acuity measurements. You determine that visual acuity is 20/50 in the right eye and 20/20 in the left eye. There is some conjunctival hyperemia. The pupil of the right eye seems to be peaked and pointing to the 7-o'clock position of the limbus. There is a small, dark, slightly

elevated body at the 7-o'clock position of the limbus. You cannot see fundus details of the right eye, but the left eye appears normal. Which of the following would be the appropriate initial management for this situation?

a. Irrigation of the limbal foreign body
b. Application of a protective shield
c. Removal of the limbal foreign body with a cotton-tipped applicator
d. Removal of the limbal foreign body using forceps
e. A prescription for topical anesthetic (eg, proparacaine 0.5%) to re-lieve the patient's symptoms, with strict instructions that he return to see you if his blurred vision continues into the week

Answer: b. Any patient whose recent activities involve striking metal on metal should be suspected of having a foreign body, even with minimal signs and symptoms. However, the case illustrated includes a giveaway sign, namely, peaking of the pupil toward the 7-o'clock position. At that position, the dark body is likely to be iris or ciliary body rather than a foreign body. This indicates a penetrating ocular injury, and the patient should be protected from further eye trauma by a protective shield. A CT scan will confirm the diagnosis of ocular or orbital foreign body. The patient should be considered an urgent referral to an ophthalmologist.

3. While cutting his roses, a neighbor develops a sudden pain in his left eye. Inspection is limited because his eyes are closed, but nothing is vis-ible on external examination.

A. What do you think might have happened?

Answer: Possibilities include a foreign body on the eye or under the lid; a superficial abrasion; or, less likely but still possible, perforation by a thorn.

B. What steps would you need to take to assess and treat this problem?

Answer: (1) Open the lids gently; never force them open, and never apply pressure to the globe if perforation is suspected. Instill a drop of topical anesthetic, if necessary, to facilitate examination. (2) Inspect the cornea and the sclera for a foreign body or possible perforation. (3) Evert the lids to look for a foreign body, unless perforation is suspected. (4) Remove the foreign body by irrigation or with a cotton-tipped applicator. (5) Act on any indications for drops, ointment, or patching. (6) If by history a possibility of ocular penetration exists, referral to an ophthalmologist is indicated. Clinical findings in such cases can be very subtle. Ocular penetration with vegetable matter such as a thorn carries not only the usual risks of ocular penetration (ie, endophthalmitis, cataract, and corneal scar) but also the possibility of a fungal infection.

4. While you are on duty in the emergency center, a patient is brought in who has been involved in a car accident. His face is bloody, especially around the eyes. His history is unclear.

A. What would you do? What would you avoid?

Answer: Cleanse carefully. Avoid pressure of any kind on the eye.

B. While cleansing, you find a cut in the eyelid. It seems easy to stitch, but the lids are swollen and the patient cannot open his eye. What next? Do you stitch the lid?

Answer: First, inspect the eye for possible perforation. Because the lid laceration is not an emergency, stitching is not immediately necessary.

C. If the eye is normal, how should you analyze the problem of the lid laceration?

Answer: The appropriate choice of treatment depends on the level of damage. If only the skin is involved, you may be able to stitch the lid. If the laceration is full-thickness or involves the lid margin, referral to an ophthalmologist is preferred. Any involvement of the canaliculi requires exquisite repair in order to avoid a tearing problem for the rest of the patient's life; referral to an ophthalmologist is mandatory.

5. A 25-year-old man visits the emergency room complaining of decreased vision and pain in his right eye after being involved in a fist fight. Although he has edema and ecchymosis of the eyelids, you are able to examine his eye. His visual acuity is 20/70 OD and 20/20 OS, and his pupils are round and reactive. However, the right pupil is sluggish, and shining a light in either eye causes pain in his right eye. He has no restriction of motility. On examination of the anterior segment, you notice a diffuse haze in the anterior chamber and early layering of blood inferiorly. Direct ophthalmoscopy is difficult, but the central retina appears flat without hemorrhages. Which of the following would be the most appropriate treatment?
   a. Instill antibiotic ointment and cycloplegic drops, apply a pressure patch, and have the patient follow up with an ophthalmologist in a few days.
   b. Prescribe steroid drops and cycloplegic drops, and tell the patient to keep his head elevated at all times.
   c. Immediately refer the patient to an ophthalmologist to rule out ruptured globe or increased intraocular pressure.

Answer: c. Although option *b* may represent appropriate treatment for hyphema, the patient needs to be adequately evaluated for a ruptured globe. The periphery of the retina needs to be evaluated closely. Option *a* represents treatment for corneal abrasion, not hyphema.

Annotated Resources

Deutsch TA, Feller DB, eds: *Paton and Goldberg's Management of Ocular Injuries.* 2nd ed. Philadelphia: WB Saunders Co; 1985. Used widely by ophthalmology residents, this book contains extensive information useful to the student or emergency center physician who desires more information on serious eye trauma.

External Disease and Cornea. Section 8 of Basic and Clinical Science Course. San Francisco: American Academy of Ophthalmology; updated annually. An excellent summary of anterior segment trauma, covering general principles, burns, superficial injuries, blunt trauma, and perforating injuries.

Kaiser PK, Corneal Abrasion Patching Study Group: A comparison of pressure patching versus no patching for corneal abrasions due to trauma or foreign body removal. *Ophthalmology* 102;12:1936–1942. Patients with noninfected non–contact-lens-related traumatic corneal abrasions and abrasions secondary to foreign body removal healed faster with less pain using antibiotics and mydriatics alone, without the need for a pressure patch.

Kaiser PK, Pineda R, Corneal Abrasion Patching Study Group: A study of topical nonsteroidal anti-inflammatory drops and no pressure patching in the treatment of corneal abrasions. *Ophthalmology* 104;8: 1353–1359. The addition of a topical NSAID to antibiotic treatment of non–contact-lens-related traumatic corneal abrasions increased patient comfort and sped time to resumption of normal activities.

Newell FW: *Ophthalmology: Principles and Concepts.* 8th ed. St Louis: CV Mosby Co; 1996. Ocular injuries are summarized succinctly in "Injuries of the Eye" in this comprehensive textbook.

Trobe JD: *The Physician's Guide to Eye Care.* San Francisco: American Academy of Ophthalmology; 1993. A brief but comprehensive resource covering the principal clinical ophthalmic problems that nonophthalmologist physicians are likely to encounter, organized for practical use by practitioners.

Chapter 6

Amblyopia and Strabismus

Objectives

As a primary care physician, you should be able to recognize the signs and symptoms of amblyopia and strabismus; be able to perform the necessary tests to screen for these conditions; and, if the patient is a child, be cognizant of the need to arrange for prompt ophthalmologic consultation, particularly when intraocular disease is suspected.

To achieve these objectives, you should learn

- To measure or estimate visual acuity in children
- To detect strabismus by general inspection, the corneal light reflex test, and the cover test
- To perform ophthalmoscopy in a child to rule out any organic causes of impaired vision when amblyopia is suspected
- To explain to parents the need for prompt treatment of amblyopia

Relevance

Amblyopia is a form of treatable visual loss found in approximately 2% of the young adult population of the United States. It can be defined as a loss of visual acuity not correctable by glasses in an otherwise healthy eye. Amblyopia develops in infancy or early childhood and usually can be detected in very young patients, principally by measuring or estimating visual acuity. If detected and treated early, amblyopia can be cured. For best results, treatment should begin before age 5; treatment for amblyopia is rarely successful if initiated past age 10. At least half of all patients with amblyopia also have strabismus, a misalignment of the two eyes.

The pediatrician or family physician will most likely be the first to see a young patient with amblyopia or strabismus and, therefore, will have the principal responsibility for screening. The child's physician must be familiar with the different kinds of amblyopia and strabismus, the close relationship of these two conditions, and how best to detect them.

Basic Information

Vision is a developmental sensory function. Vision at birth is relatively poor, but through proper visual stimulation in the early months and years of life, a normal acuity is achieved at approximately 3 years of age. If this developmental process—the stimulation of the vision-receptive cells in the brain—is prevented because of strabismus, abnormal refractive error, congenital cataract, or some other condition, vision will not develop properly. This is a failure of the developmental process, not primarily an organic abnormality of the eye.

Amblyopia

Amblyopia results from a disruption of the normal development of vision, which distinguishes it from vision loss resulting directly from organic ocular defects, such as cataract, retinoblastoma (a life-threatening tumor of early childhood), and other inflammatory and congenital ocular disorders. It is usually unilateral, but it can (rarely) affect both eyes. Amblyopia does not cause learning disorders.

Amblyopia may develop in young children who receive visual information from one eye that is blurred or conflicts with information from the other eye. To understand how amblyopia may develop in this way, consider that the brain is receiving two stimuli for each visual event: one from a visually aligned (fixating) eye and one from an "abnormal" eye (vision blurred or eye misaligned on another target). The child's brain selects the better image and suppresses the blurred or conflicting image, which results in the faulty development of vision in the amblyopic eye. In other words, the brain continually "favors" the eye with better vision, to the eventual detriment of visual development in the other eye. For this reason, amblyopia is often referred to colloquially as "lazy eye."

A number of predisposing factors can lead to the development of amblyopia. These are summarized below.

Strabismic Amblyopia

A child can develop amblyopia in the context of strabismus (misaligned eyes). An adult onset of strabismus generally will cause diplopia (double vision) because the two eyes are not aligned on the same object. The brain of a child, on the other hand, is more adaptive. In a similar strabismic situation, the child's brain ignores (suppresses) the image from one of the eyes—usually the one that provides the blurrier image. Although such an adaptation overcomes the troublesome symptom of diplopia, this cortical suppression of sensory input from one eye may interrupt the normal development of vision in the higher centers of the brain; this interruption may result in reduced vision, which is amblyopia.

Sometimes the degree of misalignment between the two eyes is very slight, making detection of strabismus and suspicion of strabismic amblyopia difficult. Even with a small angle of strabismus, amblyopia may be quite dense.

Refractive Amblyopia

Amblyopia can result from a difference in refractive error between the two eyes. The eye with the lesser refractive error provides the clearer image and usually is favored over the other eye; suppression occurs and amblyopia develops. Children with asymmetric hyperopia are susceptible, because unequal accommodation is impossible; the child can bring only one eye at a time into focus. Refractive amblyopia may be as severe as that found in strabismic amblyopia. However, the pediatrician or family physician may overlook the possibility of amblyopia because there is no obvious strabismus. Detection of amblyopia must be based on an abnormality found in visual acuity testing.

Form-Deprivation and Occlusion Amblyopia

Form-deprivation amblyopia (amblyopia ex anopsia) can result when opacities of the ocular media, such as cataracts or corneal scarring, prevent adequate sensory input and, thus, disrupt visual development. The amblyopia can persist even when the cause of the media opacity is removed. Rarely, occlusion amblyopia can result from patching of the normal eye.

Strabismus

Strabismus is a misalignment of the two eyes, so that both eyes cannot be directed toward the object of regard. Strabismus may cause or be caused by the absence of binocular vision; as with amblyopia, strabismus does not cause learning disabilities.

It is clinically useful to distinguish between concomitant (nonparalytic) and incomitant (paralytic or restrictive) strabismus. Additionally, a number of terms are used to describe and classify strabismus. These distinctions and terms are summarized below.

Concomitant Strabismus

Strabismus is called *concomitant* or *nonparalytic* when the angle (or degree) of misalignment is approximately equal in all directions of gaze (Slide 53). The individual extraocular muscles are functioning normally, but the two eyes are simply not directed toward the same target. Most concomitant

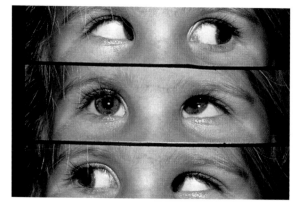

Slide 53   Concomitant strabismus. In the three views presented here, the misaligned eyes exhibit approximately the same degree of inward deviation (esotropia) in each position of gaze.

strabismus has its onset in childhood. In children, it often causes the secondary development of suppression to overcome double vision and thus leads to strabismic amblyopia. Concomitant strabismus in patients under age 6 is rarely caused by serious neurologic disease. Strabismus arising later in life may have a specific and serious neurologic basis. Concomitant strabismus may occur in an adult who loses most or all of the vision in one eye from intraocular or optic nerve disease. A blind eye in an adult will frequently drift outward, while in a child the eye will turn inward.

Incomitant Strabismus

Strabismus is called *incomitant, paralytic,* or *restrictive* when the degree of misalignment varies with the direction of gaze (Slide 54). One or more of the extraocular muscles or nerves may not be functioning properly, or normal movement may be mechanically restricted. This type of strabismus may well indicate either a serious neurologic disorder, such as third cranial nerve paresis (see Chapter 7), or an orbital disease or trauma, such as the restrictive ophthalmopathy of thyroid disease or a blowout fracture.

Heterophoria and Heterotropia

Heterophoria is a latent tendency for misalignment of the two eyes that becomes manifest only if binocular vision is interrupted, such as by covering one eye. During binocular viewing, the two eyes of a patient with heterophoria are aligned perfectly; both eyes are directed at the same object of regard. However, when one eye is covered, that eye will drift to its position of rest. Once the cover is removed, the eye will realign itself with the other eye. A minor degree of heterophoria is normal for most individuals.

Heterotropia is really another term for strabismus. In general, *tropia* refers to a manifest deviation that is present when both eyes are open (no covers). Usually, binocular vision is reduced. Some patients, however, can demonstrate an intermittent heterotropia and thus achieve binocular vision part of the time.

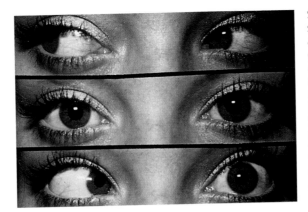

Slide 54 Incomitant strabismus. The eyes appear straight in right gaze (top) and straight-ahead gaze (middle), but a misalignment is obvious in left gaze (bottom), indicating a paralysis of the left lateral rectus muscle or a restriction of the left medial rectus. These eye positions would be found in a left sixth cranial nerve palsy.

Heterotropia and heterophoria can be subdivided further according to the direction of the deviation involved. In esotropia and esophoria, the deviating eye is directed inward toward the nose. Esotropia is a manifest deviation and is the most common type of deviation in childhood. Exotropia is much more likely to be intermittent than esotropia, with an outward deviation of an eye alternating with alignment of the eyes. Children with this condition suppress double vision when the deviating eye is turned out and achieve some degree of binocular vision when the two eyes are straight. Vertical heterotropias and heterophorias have many different causes, including paralysis or dysfunction of vertically acting extraocular muscles. When vertical deviations are described, the deviating eye (right or left) should be specified. Table 6.1 summarizes the directions of deviation in heterophoria and heterotropia. Figure 6.1 depicts the different kinds of heterotropia.

How to Examine and Interpret the Findings

Pediatric vision screening is important for detecting not only amblyopia and strabismus but also congenital cataract, glaucoma, retinoblastoma, and other vision- or life-threatening conditions. Regular screening by the pediatrician or family physician helps ensure that the child's vision is developing normally or, if it is not, that early treatment is instituted. At a minimum, all children should undergo an evaluation to detect eye and vision abnormalities during the first few months of life and again at about 3 years.

Visual acuity testing is important for detecting amblyopia as well as refractive error, which can lead to amblyopia in young children. Strabismus may be detected by general inspection, the corneal light reflex test, or the cover test. Additional tests are important for general eye screening in children of all ages: pupillary reactions are important in assessing normal eye function and health; direct ophthalmoscopy is required to detect media opacities by eliciting a red reflex and to examine the fundus for retinal abnormalities. These techniques are discussed later in the chapter.

Table 6.1   Summary of Heterophoria and Heterotropia

Prefix	Name of Disorder		Description
	-phoria (latent)	-tropia (manifest)	
eso-	esophoria	esotropia	inward deviation
exo-	exophoria	exotropia	outward deviation
hyper-	hyperphoria	hypertropia	upward deviation
hypo-	hypophoria	hypotropia	downward deviation

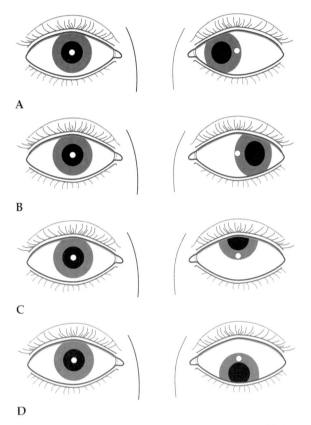

Figure 6.1 Types of heterotropia. Note the corneal light reflex. (**A**) Esotropia (inward). (**B**) Exotropia (outward). (**C**) Hypertropia (upward). (**D**) Hypotropia (downward).

Amblyopia Testing

Amblyopia can be detected by testing the visual acuity in each eye separately. Although there is no specific Mendelian pattern of inheritance, strabismus and amblyopia cluster in families. Restoration of normal visual acuity can be successful only if treatment is instituted during the first decade of life, when the visual system is still in the formative stage. Techniques for measuring or estimating visual acuity (or visual function) and detecting amblyopia vary with the child's age, as described below.

Newborns

True visual acuity cannot be measured in newborns. However, infants' general ocular status should be assessed through corneal light reflex testing, evaluation of the red reflex, pupillary testing, and, if possible, fundus examination.

Infants to 2-Year-Olds

With infants, it is possible only to assess visual function, not visual acuity. To test for amblyopia in infants (from a few months to about 2 years old), cover each eye in turn with the hand or, preferably, an adhesive patch and note how the child reacts. The infant should be able to maintain central fixation with each eye. If amblyopia is present, the child will likely protest—vocally or by evasive movements—the covering of the "good" eye. Visual function, including ocular motility, may be further assessed by passing an interesting object, such as a ring of keys, before the baby and noting how the infant watches and follows the moving object. Moving the child's head can be used to demonstrate full ocular motility if not otherwise documented by following movements.

Age 2 to 4 or 5

A picture card (Figure 6.2) may be used to test visual acuity in children between 2 and 3 years old. At age 3 (or before, if the child can follow directions and communicate adequately), visual acuity should be tested with the tumbling E chart (Figure 6.3). Use of an adhesive patch is the best way to ensure full monocular occlusion and accurate acuity measurement in children at these ages.

Vision should be rechecked annually once visual acuity has been determined to be normal in each eye. Young children may not quite reach 20/20 acuity; this is no cause for concern as long as vision is at least 20/40 and both eyes are equal.

Age 4 or 5 and Up

The Snellen chart may be used to test visual acuity in children aged 4 or 5 and up who know the letters of the alphabet (see Chapter 1). A recent

NEAR VISION TEST

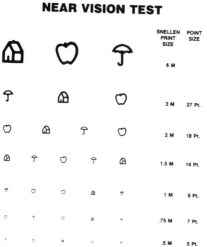

Figure 6.2   Picture card. This figure shows one type of picture card used to test visual acuity in young children. To use the picture card, the examiner familiarizes the child with the pictures at close range. Each eye is then tested individually at a testing distance of 6 meters (20 feet) from the child by asking the child to name the various objects.

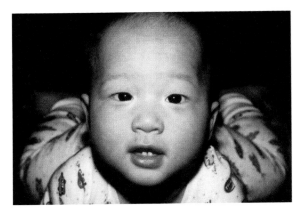

Figure 6.3   Tumbling E chart. Visual acuity testing in children should be done at 6 meters (20 feet) with charts such as the tumbling E shown here. The child indicates the direction of the "arms" of the E by pointing with his or her fingers.

Slide 55   Epicanthus. An extended lid fold and a relatively flat nose bridge may give the false appearance of an esotropia.

advance in early detection of amblyogenic factors is photoscreening. A computerized camera takes a photograph of the child's undilated eyes. Refractive errors, strabismus, anisometropia, and media opacities are visible in the photos. This technique permits screening of preverbal children and those unable to cooperate with other types of testing.

Strabismus Testing

Strabismus testing for children (and adults) consists of general inspection, the corneal light reflex test, and the cover test, all described below.

Children up to 3 or 4 months old may exhibit temporary uncoordinated eye movements and intermittent strabismus. However, if occasional deviation persists beyond this age, a referral to an ophthalmologist should be made. Constant deviations should be referred at any age.

Epicanthus (Slide 55), in which epicanthal skin folds extend toward the upper eyelid and brow and the nose bridge is flat, may give an infant the appearance of esotropia, especially if the head or eyes are turned slightly to the right or left. As the child's head grows and the nose bridge develops, the epicanthus becomes less obvious. This may be mistakenly interpreted as the child outgrowing presumed strabismus; however, a child does not outgrow a true strabismus. The cover test and evaluation of the corneal light reflex will distinguish between pseudostrabismus (epicanthus) and true strabismus. However, it is important to keep in mind that strabismus *can* also occur in the presence of epicanthus.

General Inspection

For infants and older children, a general inspection may reveal an identifiable deviation of one eye. Having the patient look in the six cardinal positions of gaze may reveal whether the deviation is approximately the same in all fields—indicating concomitant strabismus—or is significantly different in one field of gaze—indicating a possible incomitant strabismus. Involuntary eye jerks known as *nystagmus* may be detected in primary or other fields of gaze. The patient may assume an abnormal head posture (ie, a tilt or turn to one side) to reduce the nystagmus and improve the visual

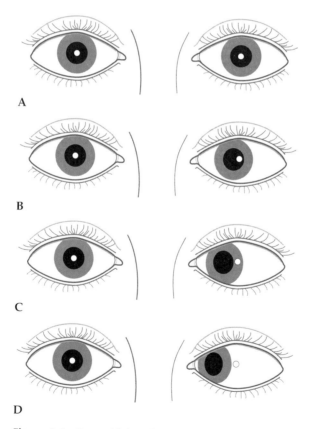

A

B

C

D

Figure 6.4 Corneal light reflex. The position of the light reflection indicates (**A**) a normal alignment, (**B**) a small esotropia, (**C**) a moderate esotropia, and (**D**) a large left esotropia.

acuity or to obtain binocular vision in cases of congenital cranial-nerve palsy. All infants or children with nystagmus should be examined and followed up by an ophthalmologist.

Corneal Light Reflex

Observation of the corneal light reflex constitutes an objective assessment of ocular alignment. Certainly in newborns and often in young children, it may be the only feasible method of testing for strabismus.

The patient is directed to look at a penlight held directly in front of the eyes by the examiner at a distance of 2 feet. The examiner aligns his or her eye with the light source and compares the position of the light as reflected by the cornea of each eye (Figure 6.4). Normally, the light is reflected on each cornea symmetrically and in the same position relative to the pupil and visual axis of each eye. In a deviating eye, the light reflection will be eccentrically positioned and in a direction opposite to that of the deviation. The size of the deviation can be estimated by the amount of displacement of the light reflex, but this is a relatively gross estimate.

Cover Test

The cover test (Figure 6.5) is easy to perform, requires no special equipment, and detects almost every case of tropia. It can be used on any patient over the age of 6 or 7 months. To perform the test, have the patient look at a fixation point, such as a detailed or interesting target (eg, a toy) or the Snellen chart. Note which eye seems to be the fixating eye. Cover the fixating eye and observe the other eye. If the uncovered eye moves to pick up

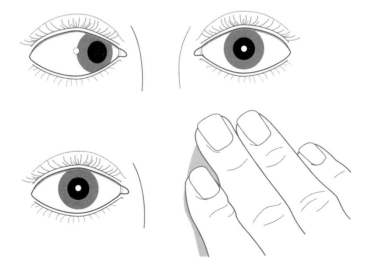

Figure 6.5 Cover test. The cover test can be used to screen for strabismus. The results depicted here indicate a right esotropia. When the left eye is covered, the right eye moves outward to pick up fixation. (When the left eye is uncovered, the left eye moves outward to pick up fixation and both eyes assume their original positions.)

the fixation, then it can be reasoned that this eye was not directed toward the object of regard originally (ie, when both eyes were uncovered). If the eye moves inward to fixate, then originally it must have been deviated outward and hence is exotropic. If the eye moves outward to fixate, then it was deviated inward and is esotropic. If the eye moves up or down, then it is hypotropic or hypertropic, respectively; the deviating eye must be specified in a hypertropia or hypotropia. Of course, each eye must be tested separately because there is no way of knowing which eye may be expressing the deviation.

No shift on cover testing means there is no tropia, but a phoria could still be present. A phoria is detected by alternate cover testing. Each eye is alternately occluded and the examiner observes the uncovered eye for a refixation shift. The patient has an esophoria if the uncovered eye moves outward to fixate, and an exophoria if the eye moves inward to fixate.

A very small-angle deviation (Slide 56) may be difficult to detect by evaluating the corneal light reflex or performing the cover test. For this reason, visual acuity testing is important in all cases of suspected strabismus for detection of amblyopia.

Other Tests

The following tests are part of general screening for all children.

Red Reflex

Light is reflected off the fundus as red when it is examined through the ophthalmoscope from a distance of about 1 foot (the red reflex; see Slide 1 in Chapter 1). Media opacities appear in the red reflex as black silhouettes (see Slide 17 in Chapter 3). Leukocoria ("white pupil"), is a white reflex that may signify the presence of cataract or retinoblastoma (Slide 57).

All infants and children should be evaluated for the red reflex; pupillary dilation may be necessary to achieve a red reflex (phenylephrine 1.0% and cyclopentolate 0.2% in infants, readily available in combination as Cyclomydril). If the examiner cannot elicit a red reflex, the infant or child should be referred to an ophthalmologist urgently.

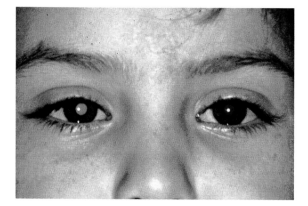

Slide 56 Small-angle right esotropia. The corneal light reflex in the right eye is displaced very slightly to the temporal aspect of the pupil.

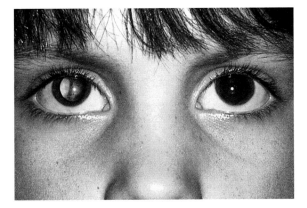

Slide 57   Leukocoria. A cataract is not the only cause of a white reflex. In this child, a retinoblastoma fills the vitreous cavity. Any change from the normal red reflex warrants careful ophthalmic examination.

Ophthalmoscopy

A careful ophthalmoscopic examination of both eyes through dilated pupils is mandatory for any patient with reduced vision or with strabismus. In this way, the examiner can detect potentially serious intraocular lesions, such as cataract, malignancies such as retinoblastoma, or other abnormalities.

Pupillary Testing

Abnormal pupillary responses may indicate neurologic disease or other ocular defects. Pupillary testing is discussed in Chapter 1; further discussion and specific techniques appear in Chapter 7.

Management or Referral

The early detection of amblyopia and strabismus is an important responsibility for those involved in infant and child health care. Delayed diagnosis may have serious consequences for visual acuity, eye disease, or systemic disease. If an abnormality is suspected, the patient should be referred promptly to an ophthalmologist.

Amblyopia

In children younger than 5, strabismic amblyopia can usually be treated effectively by the ophthalmologist through occlusion of the unaffected eye. The child wears an adhesive patch over the good eye, forcing the brain to utilize the previously suppressed eye. In general, the success of occlusion treatment for amblyopia patients between the ages of 5 and 9 will depend on the age of the patient, the degree of the amblyopia, and the persistence of patient compliance with treatment. Treatment is better tolerated by younger children but can be successful in children as old as 10. A treatment program started early in life often must be continued throughout the patient's first decade. Amblyopia treatment by patch occlusion of the unaffected eye must be monitored carefully, especially during the younger years, to avoid causing amblyopia through sensory deprivation of the occluded eye.

Treatment of refractive amblyopia consists first of wearing glasses, followed by patching of the better eye if the visual acuity difference persists after 4 to 8 weeks of wear. Equal vision in both eyes is readily achievable with parental cooperation. In general, the earlier the individual with amblyopia is diagnosed and treated, the better the chance of achieving equal vision.

Strabismus

The most effective way to support fusion (binocular vision) is to treat the amblyopia and equalize the vision. Glasses can treat some or all of the esotropia in a farsighted, or hyperopic, individual and may decrease the frequency of deviation in a myopic individual with exotropia. However, surgical correction of the misalignment may still be necessary, particularly in those children who develop esotropia before the age of 6 months (congenital esotropia). Even when binocular vision may not be achievable, the impact of a disfiguring strabismus on a patient's self-image is a valid indication for surgery. It must be stressed that surgery is not an alternative to glasses and patching when amblyopia is present.

Optometric "vision training" is rarely indicated for the treatment of amblyopia or strabismus.

Points to Remember

1. Amblyopia must be detected early to be treated successfully.
2. The importance of visual acuity testing in detecting amblyopia cannot be overemphasized. Amblyopia may be present in eyes without strabismus, so the vision in each eye may not be normal even if the eyes appear normally aligned.
3. Several serious organic conditions cause strabismus as one manifestation of the disease; therefore, all patients with strabismus should be referred to an ophthalmologist at the time of diagnosis for further testing.
4. Children may have cataracts, glaucoma, and retinal diseases, so children with unusually large eye(s), decreased or no red reflex, or poor vision should be referred to an ophthalmologist.

Sample Problems

1. A 3-year-old boy is brought to you by his mother, who tells you that she suspects his right eye is not straight. What steps would you take to determine if a significant problem is present?

Answer: Visual acuity testing should be attempted using the tumbling E chart or a picture card, with each eye alternately covered by an adhesive patch. A difference in visual acuity between the eyes or decreased vision in both eyes is significant.

Test the alignment of the eyes by evaluating the corneal light reflex. Then proceed to the cover test. Unequal positioning of the light reflex or movement of the uncovered eye to pick up the fixation would suggest a misalignment of the eyes.

Perform an ophthalmoscopic examination, preferably through dilated pupils, to determine if there is any intraocular basis for visual loss, such as cataract, retinoblastoma, or a retinal abnormality.

If visual acuity is asymmetric or if there is a suspicion of intraocular disease, the patient should be referred for an urgent ophthalmologic evaluation. If visual acuity and the fundus examination are normal but strabismus is suspected because of other examination findings or patient history, a nonurgent referral should be made.

2. A family has just moved into your area and the mother brings her 6-month-old baby to your family practice office for a routine checkup. She mentions that the child's grandfather has noted that in several photographs the baby's left eye appears crossed. He is adamant in his observation and feels that "something should be done." The mother has felt that, at times, the eye has appeared crossed, but the baby's father has not observed this phenomenon. How should you proceed?

Answer: Inquire about any family history of strabismus or amblyopia and evaluate for the presence of epicanthus. Place your hand in front of one eye and then the other to see if the child exhibits displeasure. Observe the alignment of the child's eyes as well as extraocular movements if possible. Use a penlight to assess the position of the corneal light reflex.

Examination reveals that significant lid folds are present. The corneal light reflex is the same in each eye, and full extraocular movements are seen in all cardinal fields of gaze. Although in this case the appearance of a crossed eye is probably the result of epicanthus, continued observation on the next visit is indicated. Remember that strabismus and amblyopia can occur in a patient with epicanthus, and the strabismus may be intermittent. Any suspected abnormality should be referred to an ophthalmologist.

3. A 2-year-old boy is brought to your office because his mother has noticed that over the past 2 weeks his right eye has deviated inward during periods of fatigue. On the previous evening, the boy's father claimed to have noted a white reflex in the child's right eye. How should you proceed?

Answer: Show the child a toy and cover his left eye with your hand; evaluate his response. Cover his right eye to compare his response. Evaluate the corneal light reflex and perform the cover test. In particular, note whether an abnormal response is elicited on covering one eye.

Test the pupillary light reflexes. Perform an ophthalmoscopic examination, preferably through a dilated pupil, to assess the red reflex and observe for organic pathology.

Examination reveals equal pupillary light reflexes. A white reflex is noted on ophthalmoscopic examination of the right eye as compared with the left. No detail can be seen in the right fundus. Your findings indicate the need for an urgent referral. Following ophthalmologic consultation, the esotropia in this child was diagnosed as secondary to a retinoblastoma.

4. A 54-year-old man has early cataracts in both eyes. With glasses, the right eye cannot be corrected to better than 20/200, whereas with the left eye he can read the 20/40 line with best correction. The amount of cataract is exactly the same in each eye. Examination of the optic disc and macula, pupillary reaction, color vision, and retinal blood vessels proved entirely normal in each eye. However, the right eye appears to be turned slightly inward when you evaluate the corneal light reflex, and the patient has not experienced diplopia. Additional questioning reveals that the patient wore a patch over one eye as a child. Why would information concerning his childhood ocular condition be relevant in this situation?

   Answer: The poor vision in the right eye may be due to a long-standing amblyopia. If this is the case, an ophthalmologist will conclude that removal of the cataract would result in vision only as good as that during the adolescent years and surgery would probably not be recommended.

5. A 4-year-old boy with attention-deficit disorder comes to your office for his routine preschool physical examination. Your nurse tests his visual acuity with the picture card and obtains 20/30 vision on the right. During testing of the left eye the patient loses attention and refuses to cooperate further with testing. What course of action should you take?

   Answer: Often children become uncooperative with visual acuity testing due to poor vision in the eye being tested. This is sometimes misinterpreted as a behavioral rather than an ocular issue. This patient can return on another day to have the left eye tested first, with the right eye covered by an adhesive patch. If visual acuity measurement is still unsuccessful, the patient should be referred to an ophthalmologist for evaluation.

6. A 4-year-old girl is brought to your office by her mother, who says that she sees her daughter's right eye "drifting." You test the patient's vision, which is 20/20 in each eye. There is no epicanthus. The corneal light test shows no deviation, and the cover test fails to reveal strabismus. What is your next step?

   Answer: Strabismus can be intermittent. Intermittent esodeviations are usually early manifestations of a constant deviation and may be difficult to detect during the early stages. Intermittent exodeviations are more pronounced when the patient is tired or sick but can be easily missed. If the patient has a reliable history of strabismus but you are unable to detect the deviation, referral to an ophthalmologist is recommended.

7. A mother reports that her 1-year-old child is sensitive to light and his right eye looks larger than the left. On examination you note that although the child's right eye does look larger, the pupillary reactions are equal in both eyes, the corneas are clear, and there is a good red reflex in each eye. What should you tell the mother?
   a. Do not worry, the child will "grow into" his eyes.
   b. Return in 1 month for a reexamination.
   c. Take the child to an ophthalmologist on my referral.
   d. This is probably a cancer of the right eye, and you should take the child to an oncologist on my referral.

   Answer: c. Children can have glaucoma, which causes buphthalmos, or enlargement of one or both eyes. Although glaucoma may be associated with increased tearing, sensitivity to light, and a hazy or white cornea, the only sign of glaucoma in some children may be enlargement of the eye or eyes. This child should be referred immediately to an ophthalmologist for diagnosis and management.

Annotated Resources

Gittinger JW Jr: *Ophthalmology: A Clinical Introduction*. Boston: Little, Brown & Co; 1984:131–149. Provides the reader with a concise overview of strabismus and amblyopia. A short section on the anatomy and function of the extraocular muscles is particularly good.

Newell FW: *Ophthalmology: Principles and Concepts*. 8th ed. St Louis: CV Mosby Co; 1996. Disorders of ocular motility are well covered. The short discussion of the development of amblyopia will be beneficial to the reader. Ocular muscle function and ocular motility are presented in different areas of the textbook. Provides a good overview.

Trobe JD: *The Physician's Guide to Eye Care*. San Francisco: American Academy of Ophthalmology; 1993. A brief but comprehensive resource covering the principal clinical ophthalmic problems that nonophthalmologist physicians are likely to encounter, organized for practical use by practitioners.

Vaughan DG, Asbury T, Riordan-Eva P: *General Ophthalmology*. 14th ed. Norwalk, CT: Appleton & Lange; 1995. The chapter on strabismus is a well-illustrated, comprehensive review of the subject.

Chapter 7

Neuro-Ophthalmology

Objectives

As a primary care physician, you should be able to perform a basic neuro-ophthalmic examination and to recognize and interpret the more common signs and symptoms of neuro-ophthalmic disorders.

To achieve these objectives, you should learn

- To measure visual acuity
- To examine pupillary reactions
- To test the function of the extraocular muscles
- To evaluate the visual fields
- To inspect the optic nerve head

Relevance

The visual pathways and the oculomotor system reflect much of the status of the nervous system as a whole. Approximately 35% of the sensory fibers entering the brain are in the two optic nerves. It is estimated that 65% of intracranial diseases exhibit neuro-ophthalmic symptoms or signs. Routine neurovisual examination allows the primary care physician to identify abnormalities indicating life-threatening or vision-threatening neurologic disorders and other systemic diseases. Important examples are brain tumors, multiple sclerosis, cerebrovascular disease, giant-cell arteritis, and intracranial arterial aneurysms.

How to Examine

The neuro-ophthalmic survey may be simplified to the point where only a few minutes of the primary care physician's time are required, or a detailed neuro-ophthalmic examination may occupy many hours of an ophthalmologist's time and need to be substantiated by sophisticated procedures. This chapter will address routine tests and screening procedures.

Visual Acuity Testing

The first step in any eye examination is to measure visual acuity in each eye. The chief complaint of most patients with ocular problems is some aberration of vision. Measurement of visual acuity is an absolute necessity. Use of the conventional Snellen eye chart is currently the easiest and best method of measuring the function of the macular fibers, although any reading material may be useful for screening purposes. Both distance and near vision ideally should be measured and recorded using the patient's corrective lenses if available. (See Chapter 1 for performance instructions.)

Visual Field Testing

Evaluation of the visual fields should never be omitted from the basic eye examination. Gross confrontation field testing is an accepted screening procedure. Each eye must be tested separately. While fixing on the examiner's eye with the nonoccluded eye, the patient is asked to count fingers in each of the four quadrants of the visual field. (See Chapter 1 for a detailed description of confrontation field testing.)

Because most visual field defects affect central vision, attention should be paid to the area within the central 30°. A method of screening for central field defects is to ask the patient to look at a piece of graph paper or an Amsler grid, which is similar but specific for this type of testing. (See Figure 3.4 in Chapter 3 for a depiction of the Amsler grid and further discussion on its use in central visual field testing.) Sometimes, use of a grid will demonstrate subtle bitemporal hemianopic field loss due to chiasmal compression or small homonymous field defects due to occipital lobe disease. An acceptable alternative method includes asking the patient to recognize a small, white pin head or similar object in all fields of vision. A red test object may also be valuable in evaluating patients with optic nerve or chiasmal disease.

Pupillary Reactions

Pupils should be inspected while the patient is looking at distance to avoid the pupillary constriction that occurs with a near target. Inspection of pupils in patients with dark-brown irides can be facilitated with a tangentially applied light. The pupils should be round and equal in diameter, although less than 1 millimeter of inequality may be a normal variation. Poor pupillary dilation in dim light may indicate dysfunction of the sympathetic nervous system, and poor pupillary constriction to bright light may indicate parasympathetic dysfunction. For schematic illustrations of the pupillary pathways and reflexes, see Figures 7.1 and 7.2.

The swinging-flashlight test is the most valuable clinical test for optic nerve dysfunction currently available to the general physician. The abnormality detected with this test is the afferent pupillary defect, also known as the Marcus Gunn pupil (see "Afferent Defect" in Figure 7.2). To perform

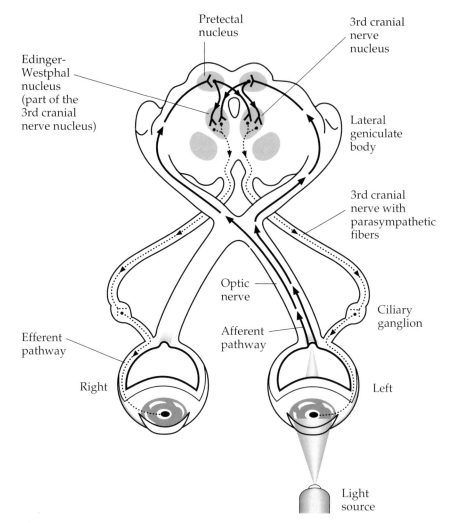

Figure 7.1 Pupillary pathways. The view shown is a cross-section. The dotted line represents the efferent pathway, and the solid line represents the afferent pathway. A light stimulating the left retina will generate impulses that travel up the left optic nerve and divide at the chiasm. Some impulses continue up the left tract; some cross and continue up the right tract. The impulses arrive at each pretectal nucleus and stimulate cells, which in turn send impulses down the third cranial nerve to each iris sphincter, causing each pupil to contract. It is because of the double decussation, the first in the chiasm and the second between the pretectal nuclei and the Edinger-Westphal nuclei, that the direct pupil response in the left eye equals the consensual response in the right eye.

this test, dim room illumination and a bright light are helpful. The patient maintains fixation on an object 15 feet or more away. The bright light is held directly in front of one eye for 3 to 5 seconds, moved rapidly across the bridge of the nose to the front of the other eye for 3 to 5 seconds, and then shifted back to the first eye. This procedure should be repeated several times until the examiner is certain of the responses. The critical observation to be made is the behavior of the pupil when it is first illuminated.

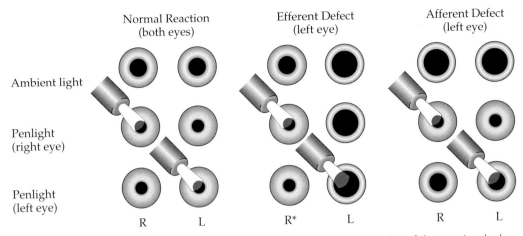

Normal Reaction (both eyes) Efferent Defect (left eye) Afferent Defect (left eye)

Ambient light

Penlight (right eye)

Penlight (left eye)

R L R* L R L

Figure 7.2 Pupillary reflexes. The orientation depicted is that of the examiner looking at the patient's eyes.
*Note normal constriction from consensual response.

A normal response is initial pupillary constriction followed by variable amounts of redilation. An abnormal response is slow dilation without initial constriction. The relative afferent pupillary defect almost always indicates a lesion in the optic nerve on the affected side, although rarely a large retinal lesion may produce this defect. Additional support for the diagnosis may be gained by asking the patient to compare the brightness of the light or the color of a red object between the two eyes. A patient with an optic neuropathy will usually say that the light does not appear as bright and that a red object appears faded with the eye that has an afferent pupillary defect.

Ocular Motility Testing

Eye movements should be tested, especially if the patient has a complaint of double vision or if any neurologic disease is suspected. First, alignment of the eyes should be assessed to identify a deviation that could be due to strabismus, extraocular muscle malfunction, or oculomotor nerve dysfunction. (See "Ocular Motility Testing" in Chapter 1 and "Strabismus Testing" in Chapter 6.) Ophthalmoplegia can be distinguished from non-paralytic strabismus by the presence of incomitancy. Rapid eye movements (saccades) are tested by asking the patient to direct the eyes quickly to a target that the examiner is holding right, left, up, and down. Tracking movements (pursuit) are tested by asking the patient to follow a slowly moving target first horizontally and then vertically. The examiner should be looking for the following abnormalities:

1. Strabismus
2. Limitation of movement of one eye
3. Limitation of gaze (both eyes affected similarly)
4. Nystagmus (spontaneous jerking eye movements)

Ophthalmoscopy

Evaluation of a patient with neurologic symptoms is not complete without evaluation of the ocular fundus. Particular attention should be given to the appearance of the optic disc. In some neuro-ophthalmic conditions, the optic disc may be swollen and elevated; in others, it may be pale and atrophic. The examiner should attempt to note the presence of spontaneous venous pulsations, indicating that the intracranial pressure is normal (not elevated).

How to Interpret the Findings

Pupillary Disorders

Disorders of pupillary function are among the most accurate of the localizing signs of neurologic disease. Ocular disease and the influence of systemic or local drugs on the pupils must be assessed before pupillary abnormalities can be considered neurologically significant. Some commonly encountered pupillary abnormalities are discussed below.

Dilated Pupil

A dilated pupil, especially one that does not react to light, usually indicates a lesion in the efferent limb of the pupillary reflex (see "Efferent Defect" in Figure 7.2). A dilated pupil in a patient with a head injury or a cloudy sensorium may indicate compression of the third cranial nerve (oculomotor nerve) by herniation of the temporal lobe and may have grave importance. A life-threatening aneurysm also can manifest with a dilated pupil, usually associated with a droopy lid and double vision. On the other hand, a dilated, fixed pupil in an otherwise asymptomatic, healthy patient is usually benign. In a healthy individual, a dilated pupil may reflect a benign lesion in the ciliary ganglion (an Adie's tonic pupil) or may be secondary to instillation of a dilating eyedrop or use of certain motion-sickness medications.

Tonic Pupil

The tonic pupil, known as *Adie's pupil*, is seen predominantly in young women and is usually unilateral. In ordinary light, the tonic pupil is usually larger than its counterpart; the reaction to light is either diminished or absent. Instillation of weak cholinergic agents (eg, 1/8% pilocarpine hydrochloride) will cause constriction of a tonic pupil, indicating denervation hypersensitivity, whereas this constriction will not occur in a normal pupil. By itself, a tonic pupil is of no neurologic significance.

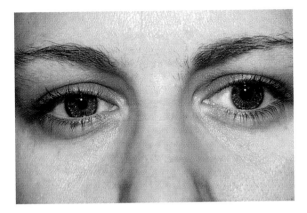

Slide 58   Horner's syndrome. This acquired lesion of the cervical sympathetic chain has caused a mild ptosis of the right upper eyelid and a narrowing of the right pupil.

Unilateral Small Pupil

A small pupil in one eye that has normal reactivity to light and near stimuli is usually physiologic and is of no neurologic significance. However, when accompanied by ptosis of the upper eyelid, a small pupil may indicate Horner's syndrome (Slide 58). Horner's syndrome is caused by a congenital or an acquired lesion of the sympathetic pathways, either in the central or preganglionic portion from the hypothalamus to the superior cervical ganglion or in the postganglionic portion from the cervical ganglion to the eye (Figure 7.3). Carotid dissection, carotid aneurysm, and tumor are life-threatening lesions that can present with Horner's syndrome. Detection of Horner's syndrome can be accomplished through the topical instillation of 4% cocaine, which will dilate a normal pupil but not a desympathectomized pupil. Differentiation of preganglionic from postganglionic lesions is important and can usually be accomplished through the instillation of hydroxyamphetamine drops if available.

Argyll Robertson pupil is a small, irregular pupil that constricts to light poorly or not at all but constricts normally to convergence. Usually both pupils are involved. However, initial involvement may be unilateral or asymmetric. Because Argyll Robertson pupil is associated with tertiary syphilis, the patient should be evaluated for syphilis with RPR or VDRL and FTA-ABS testing.

Neuromotility Disorders

Some significant oculomotor disorders that the primary care physician should recognize are discussed below. (It may be helpful to refer to Figure 1.3, which illustrates the extraocular muscles.)

Evaluation of the patient whose complaint is double vision must include a thorough, neurologically oriented history. True diplopia—which means that two separate, equally bright images are visualized, with one of the images disappearing when one eye is closed—signifies strabismus

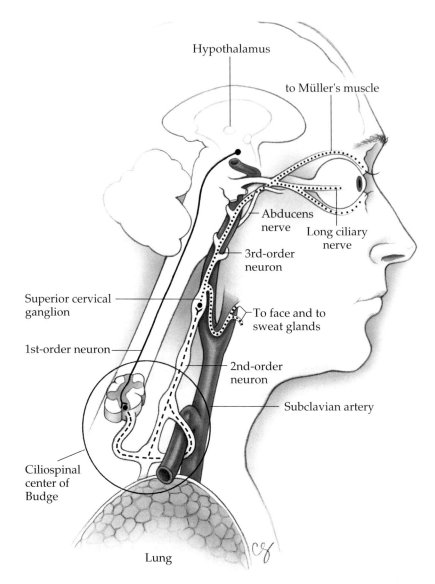

Hypothalamus

to Müller's muscle

Abducens
nerve   Long ciliary
nerve

3rd-order
neuron

Superior cervical
ganglion

To face and to
sweat glands

1st-order neuron

2nd-order
neuron

Subclavian artery

Ciliospinal
center of
Budge

Lung

Figure 7.3   Anatomy of sympathetic pathway. Shown are pathways of first-order central neuron (solid line), second-order intermediate neuron (dashed line), and third-order neuron (dotted line). Note the proximity of pulmonary apex to sympathetic chain, as well as the relationship of the intracavernous sympathetic fibers to the abducens nerve. (Illustration by Christine Gralapp.)

acquired after the age of 7 or 8 years. Patients sometimes say they have double vision when they mean they have blurred vision of one eye; for example, aberration due to corneal disease, cataract, or strands of mucus in the tear film. It is important to note in the history whether the diplopia is transient or persistent; sudden or gradual in onset; horizontal, vertical, or diagonal; and the same or different in various positions of gaze.

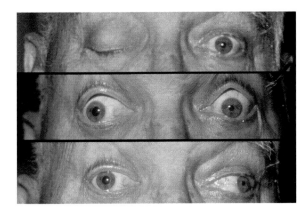

Slide 59   Third-nerve palsy. Lids are manually elevated in the middle and lower photos. Middle photo shows patient's attempt to look straight ahead; lower photo shows patient's attempt to look left.

(Reprinted by permission from Miller NR, ed: *Walsh & Hoyt's Clinical Neuro-Ophthalmology*, 4th ed, Vol 2. Baltimore: Williams & Wilkins; 1985.)

Third Cranial Nerve Paresis

Cranial nerve III (oculomotor nerve) supplies the levator palpebrae muscle of the upper eyelid, the superior rectus, medial rectus, inferior rectus, and inferior oblique muscles, as well as the parasympathetic fibers to the sphincter of the iris. Complete paralysis of the oculomotor nerve produces both horizontal and vertical diplopia, with ptosis of the upper eyelid and an inability to rotate the eye inward, upward, or downward (Slides 59 and 60). The pupil may be dilated and nonresponsive. The most common causes of isolated third-nerve palsy include intracranial aneurysm (especially of the posterior communicating artery), vaso-occlusive disease within the nerve (usually associated with diabetes and hypertension), trauma, and brain tumor.

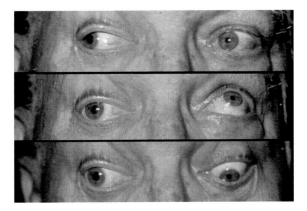

Slide 60   Third-nerve palsy. Lids are manually elevated in all photos. From top, patient's attempt to look right, up, and down.

(Reprinted by permission from Miller NR, ed: *Walsh & Hoyt's Clinical Neuro-Ophthalmology*, 4th ed, Vol 2. Baltimore: Williams & Wilkins; 1985.)

Fourth Cranial Nerve Paresis

Cranial nerve IV (trochlear nerve) innervates the superior oblique muscle so that complete paralysis causes vertical diplopia. The patient often notices more difficulty in downgaze and may tilt the head toward the opposite shoulder to minimize the diplopia. The most frequent cause of

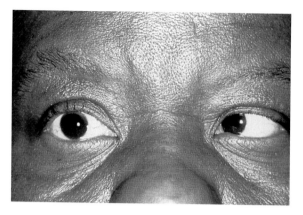

Slide 61 Sixth cranial nerve paresis. Shown here is an impairment of abduction of the right eye on right gaze.

isolated fourth-nerve palsy is closed-head trauma, but the condition is also found in patients with small-vessel disease, especially associated with hypertension or diabetes.

Sixth Cranial Nerve Paresis

Cranial nerve VI (abducens nerve) supplies the lateral rectus muscle; therefore, complete paralysis produces loss of abduction and horizontal diplopia, with the greatest separation of images in gaze directed toward the affected side (Slide 61). Intracranial tumors account for approximately 30% of cases of isolated sixth-nerve paralysis. Head trauma, small-vessel disease, viral infections, and increased intracranial pressure are also frequent causes of abducens paresis.

Other Cranial Nerve Palsies

Cranial nerve V is assessed by checking corneal sensation and bilateral facial sensation on the forehead, cheek, and chin. To reveal weakness of cranial nerve VII, ask the patient to smile and then to squeeze the eyes tightly shut, while you attempt to open the patient's eyes. To check cranial nerve VIII, ask the patient if he or she can hear the noise made as you rub your thumb and index fingertips together next to the patient's ear.

Myasthenia Gravis

Myasthenia gravis is a chronic autoimmune condition that interferes with neuromuscular transmission in skeletal muscles. The disease can affect any muscles, but ptosis and double vision are the presenting signs in about half the patients. Characterized by fatigability of muscle function on sustained effort, myasthenia gravis may mimic nearly any other oculomotor problem, including third-, fourth-, and sixth-nerve disease, gaze paresis, and internuclear ophthalmoplegia. Myasthenia gravis does not affect the pupil. All patients with unexplained diplopia or ptosis should have an edrophonium chloride (Tensilon) test.

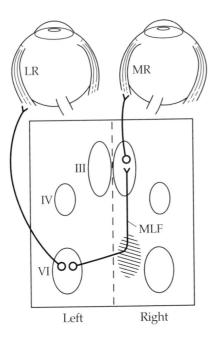

Figure 7.4 Internuclear ophthalmoplegia. Information travels from the sixth-nerve nucleus (VI) to the ipsilateral lateral rectus muscle (LR) and, via the medial longitudinal fasciculus (MLF), to the contralateral third-nerve nucleus (III) and on to the contralateral medial rectus (MR) to make both eyes turn to the side of the stimulating sixth-nerve nucleus. A lesion blocking the path between the ipsilateral sixth-nerve nucleus and the contralateral third-nerve nucleus results in an internuclear ophthalmoplegia.

Internuclear Ophthalmoplegia

Lesions of the medial longitudinal fasciculus, which carries input from the ipsilateral sixth-nerve nucleus to the contralateral third-nerve medial rectus subnucleus, are usually of considerable diagnostic significance (Figure 7.4). The clinical manifestations of such a lesion include straight eyes in primary gaze but weakness of the adducting eye and nystagmus of the abducting eye in lateral gaze (Slide 62). It may be unilateral or bilateral, and convergence is usually intact. In older individuals, unilateral internuclear ophthalmoplegia suggests small-vessel disease within the distribution of the vertebral-basilar arterial system. In young adults, bilateral internuclear ophthalmoplegia is almost always due to demyelinating disease. In children, however, internuclear ophthalmoplegia may be due to a pontine glioma.

Nystagmus

Spontaneous, rhythmic, back-and-forth movement of one or both eyes is referred to as *nystagmus* (see "General Inspection" in Chapter 6). The direction may be horizontal, vertical, rotary, or a combination.

The three most common forms of nystagmus are benign and do not indicate central nervous system dysfunction. The first form of benign nystagmus occurs in end-gaze, when the patient is attempting to maintain the eyes in extremes of lateral gaze. In this position, it is not unusual for the eyes to drift back slightly from the extreme horizontal gaze position and then refixate with a small jerk movement. End-point nystagmus is usually not well sustained and disappears as the patient is permitted to move the

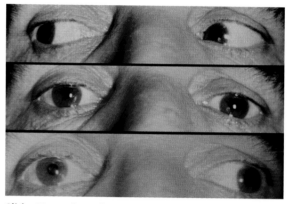

Slide 62 Unilateral right internuclear ophthalmoplegia. This 32-year-old patient with multiple sclerosis is unable to adduct the right eye on left horizontal gaze (bottom). The eyes are straight in primary gaze (middle), differentiating this condition from medial rectus underaction of intrinsic muscle or third-nerve origin.
(Reprinted by permission from Miller NR, ed: *Walsh & Hoyt's Clinical Neuro-Ophthalmology,* 4th ed, Vol 2. Baltimore: Williams & Wilkins; 1985.)

gaze slightly away from the extreme position. The second form of benign nystagmus is induced by drugs: diphenylhydantoin, barbiturates, and other sedatives. In this form, a jerk nystagmus may be present in all positions of gaze. The third form, a searching, pendular nystagmus, is commonly seen in individuals who are visually impaired from birth.

Nystagmus may indicate central nervous system dysfunction. Representative diseases that cause nystagmus are multiple sclerosis, brain tumor, and degeneration of the central nervous system.

Optic Nerve Disease

Many disorders of the anterior visual pathways are accompanied by abnormalities of the optic nerve head. These include swelling due to infiltration or inflammation or ischemia of the anterior optic nerve head and atrophy usually due to damage from various disorders.

Optic Disc Elevation

Congenital Anomalous Disc Elevation   Occurring in slightly less than 1% of the population, congenital anomalous disc elevation is a benign, nonprogressive condition. The optic disc margins are blurred, the disc substance is elevated, and the optic cup is absent. However, there is no evidence of edema or hemorrhage, and often spontaneous venous pulsation can be observed. Congenital disc elevation may be associated with hyperopia and may be accompanied by the accumulation of calcified protein within the optic disc itself (optic disc drusen). Because of its deceptive appearance, congenital fullness of the optic nerve has been referred to as *pseudopapilledema* (Slide 63, left). The condition should not be confused

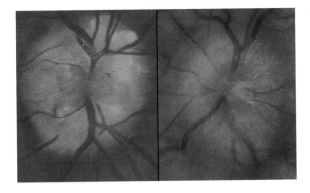

Slide 63 Pseudopapilledema and true papilledema. On the left, pseudopapilledema from optic nerve drusen is shown; note several discrete drusen on the superior edge of the disc. On the right, true papilledema is shown; note congested capillaries and swollen nerve bundles.

with true, acquired papilledema (Slide 63, right). Such differentiation may be difficult, and the diagnosis of true papilledema sometimes cannot be made without lumbar puncture, once intracranial mass has been ruled out by MRI with and without gadolinium.

Papilledema   One of the most important ophthalmoscopic findings is papilledema; swelling of the optic disc secondary to increased intracranial pressure occurs in approximately 50% of patients with a brain tumor. Characteristics of fully developed papilledema include hyperemia of the disc, tortuosity of the veins and capillaries, blurring and elevation of the margins of the disc, and hemorrhages on and surrounding the nerve head. The signs of early papilledema may not be distinct, with subtle elevation of the disc margins, loss of previously identified spontaneous venous pulsations, and mild hyperemia. In addition to intracranial mass lesions, papilledema may be seen in pseudotumor cerebri and in severe acute systemic hypertension. The first step in evaluating papilledema is to measure the blood pressure.

Papillitis   Inflammatory edema of the disc, known as *papillitis* or *anterior optic neuritis*, may be indistinguishable from papilledema by its ophthalmoscopic appearance. (For a comparison of papillitis and papilledema, see Slides 10 and 11 in Chapter 2.) Whereas papillitis is more commonly unilateral and associated with decreased visual acuity and impaired color vision, papilledema is usually bilateral and usually associated with good central vision.

Ischemic Optic Neuropathy   Ischemic optic neuropathy presents as a pale, swollen disc, often accompanied by splinter hemorrhages and loss of visual acuity and visual field. The field loss with ischemic neuropathy is often altitudinal, that is, predominantly within the superior or inferior field.

Amaurosis Fugax

Amaurosis fugax is transient monocular visual loss due to arterial insufficiency. Patients over age 50 complaining of monocular visual loss lasting several minutes should be investigated for atheroma affecting the ipsilateral carotid circulation. Atheroma may be the source of emboli that

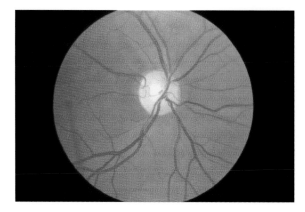

Slide 64 Optic atrophy. This disc is flat and totally white. The sharp margins and clear definition of the disc suggest a primary disturbance of the retinal ganglion cells or their axons, rather than an inflammatory cause at the disc.

transiently interrupt retinal blood flow. Evaluation of amaurosis fugax is complex, and patients should be referred to an ophthalmologist, neurologist, or vascular surgeon for further workup.

Optic Atrophy

Optic atrophy (Slide 64), or pallor of the optic disc, results from damage to the nerve fiber layer of the retina, the optic nerve itself, the optic chiasm, or the optic tracts. With progressive loss of axons and alteration in glial tissue, the optic disc becomes pale. After extensive damage, the disc may become white.

There is a wide range of normal coloration of the disc. A diagnosis of optic atrophy should not be made unless there is decreased visual acuity or visual field loss accompanying the paleness of the optic disc or, if unilateral, a relative afferent pupillary defect. Common causes of optic atrophy include

- Previous optic neuritis or long-standing papilledema
- Compression of the optic nerve by a mass lesion, such as a meningioma, or pituitary adenoma
- Ischemic damage to the optic nerve due to small-vessel disease or giant-cell arteritis
- Glaucoma (see Chapter 3)

Visual Field Defects

The following terms are commonly used to discuss visual field loss:

- **Scotoma** An area of reduced or absent vision within an otherwise intact visual field.
- **Hemianopia** Loss of half the visual field. Usually, this involves loss of either the right or the left half of the visual field in either eye; however, the term *altitudinal hemianopia* may be used to distinguish loss of the superior or inferior half of the visual field.
- **Homonymous hemianopia** Loss of either the right or the left half of the visual field in both eyes.
- **Bitemporal hemianopia** Loss of the right half of the visual field in the right eye and loss of the left half of the visual field in the left eye.

Lesions anywhere in the visual system, from the retina to the occipital lobes, will produce visual field defects (Figure 7.5). Although detection and analysis of these visual field defects have led to entire texts written on the science of perimetry, most physicians need be concerned with only a few types of visual field loss. Neurologically significant field defects are most often central scotomas (due to optic nerve lesions), bitemporal field defects (due to chiasmal disease), or homonymous visual field defects (due to retrochiasmal damage to the optic tracts, the radiations, or the occipital cortex). In almost all locations, the effects produced are most profound within the central 30° of the visual field.

Isolated lesions anterior to the chiasm within the optic nerve produce visual field defects in one eye only. Optic nerve dysfunction typically produces a central scotoma, with accompanying reduction in visual acuity. Common causes of unilateral optic neuropathy include optic neuritis, optic nerve glioma, meningioma, and ischemic optic neuropathy.

Lesions in the optic chiasm produce visual field defects that affect both eyes, but in a dissimilar fashion. The most common example is a bitemporal hemianopia caused by pituitary adenoma. Another common visual field defect due to disease near the chiasm is loss of central field in one eye and a temporal visual field defect in the other eye.

Lesions affecting the visual pathways behind the chiasm produce homonymous hemianopias or homonymous defects that are less than a complete hemianopia. Because the fibers serving the corresponding portions of the two retinas lie increasingly closer together as the fibers pass back toward the occipital cortex, there is greater correspondence of the field defects in the two eyes as the lesions occur more posteriorly. Central visual acuity is not affected in homonymous hemianopias unless both hemispheres are involved. Stroke is the most common cause of a homonymous hemianopia. Middle cerebral artery occlusion tends to cause a complete hemianopia with other neurologic signs, whereas posterior cerebral artery occlusion causes isolated, congruous (identical) hemianopic scotomas.

Points to Remember

1. Testing of both visual acuity and visual fields is critical in the evaluation of the abnormal optic disc.
2. A patient with a unilateral optic nerve lesion should have equal pupils in ambient light, but a positive swinging-flashlight test.
3. A blurred disc margin is not diagnostic for papilledema. Other signs and symptoms must be considered.
4. Chiasmal disease is most likely to cause a bitemporal field defect.
5. If one of the following is abnormal—pupil, lid position, or ocular motility—look closely for involvement of the others.
6. Cranial nerves V and VII should be checked if ocular motility is abnormal and cranial nerve palsy is suspected.
7. Slowly progressive vision loss or cranial nerve palsy should prompt consideration of a compressive lesion, such as a tumor or aneurysm.

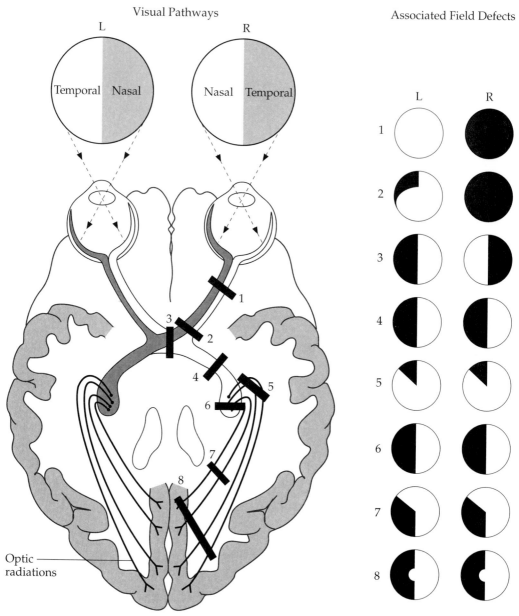

Visual Pathways

Associated Field Defects

Optic radiations

Visual cortex in occipital lobes

Figure 7.5   Visual pathways with associated field defects. For the visual pathways, the view shown is a cross-section seen from above. Note that objects in the right half of the visual field form images in the left half of each retina and are transmitted to the left hemisphere. The numbers correspond to lesions in the visual pathways and to the field defects that result from these interruptions. For the purposes of the diagram, the fields shown reflect the effects of total interruption of the indicated structures. In actuality, partial impairment is more the rule than the exception. The key at the top of the facing page indicates the site of each lesion and the associated field defect.

Figure 7.5 (continued)

Site of Lesion	Associated Field Defect
1 Optic nerve	Monocular loss of vision
2 Optic nerve merging with chiasm	Monocular loss of vision associated with contralateral impairment of temporal field
3 Optic chiasm	Bitemporal hemianopia
4 Optic tract	Total homonymous hemianopia (usually noncongruous if incomplete)
5 Temporal lobe	Upper homonymous hemianopia
6 Geniculate body	Rare total homonymous hemianopia
7 Parietal lobe	Lower homonymous quadrantanopia
8 Occipital lobe	Variety of homonymous hemianopias, ranging from total to small homonymous scotomas, depending on portion of lobe involved; high degree of congruity

Sample Problems

1. A 45-year-old woman comes to the emergency center because of severe left-sided headache and double vision that began the night before, immediately following vigorous exercise. As you examine her, she continues to complain of severe left-sided headache. Her neuro-ophthalmologic examination is normal, except that the left upper lid is ptotic; the left eye is deviated outward and fails to elevate, depress, or adduct normally; and the left pupil is dilated 3 mm more than the right and responds very poorly to light, both directly and consensually. What is your differential diagnosis? How would you proceed with evaluation and management?

   Answer: The findings are those of a left third-nerve palsy with involvement of the pupil. The features of this case—including the age and gender of the patient, the suddenness of onset, the accompanying headache, and the fact that onset occurred in conjunction with vigorous exercise—are presented to raise the issue of a possible berry aneurysm of the circle of Willis. All of the preceding factors are commonly observed in acutely expanding aneurysms arising at the junction of the internal carotid and posterior communicating arteries. Such an aneurysm is the most common cause of third-nerve palsy with pupillary involvement. Even though the patient may have no symptoms other than headache and those symptoms caused by the third-nerve palsy, an aneurysm must be suspected. This is one of the true ophthalmic emergencies. The management in this case calls for an immediate neurosurgical consultation.

   In this situation, the pupil was dilated. If the same patient appeared with exactly the same findings except for a normal left pupil, the diagnosis and management would be different. A pupil-sparing third-nerve palsy most likely is due to diabetes or some other microvascular obstruction causing ischemia of the core of the oculomotor nerve.

Therefore, a pupil-sparing third-nerve palsy is not a neurosurgical emergency and the patient should be worked up for diabetes, giant-cell arteritis, syphilis, and other vascular disease. It is important to note that a third-nerve palsy can be considered pupil-sparing only if the palsy is complete and the pupil is totally normal.

2. A 25-year-old medical student suddenly complains of horizontal diplopia. Her eyes are straight when looking directly ahead, but when she attempts to look to the right or left, the adducting eye fails to move normally. However, when she is asked to look at the examiner's finger at a distance of 6 inches, both eyes converge normally. She also exhibits vertical nystagmus when she looks up. What is the neuro-anatomic localization of this problem? What is the etiologic diagnosis?

   Answer: The description is that of bilateral internuclear ophthalmoplegia. The medial longitudinal fasciculi conduct impulses to those third cranial nerve nuclei essential for participation in horizontal gaze movements. Acute, bilateral impairment of function of the medial longitudinal fasciculi occurring in this age group is typical of multiple sclerosis.

3. A 32-year-old female geologist has noticed slowly progressive blurring of vision for about a month. An optometrist changed her prescription, but the new glasses were of minimal benefit. After the symptom had been present for 3 months, she visited her family doctor, who found nothing wrong and referred her to a neurologist. The neurologist could find no abnormality and suggested she might be suffering from stress. She has now come to the emergency center because her vision has become distressingly blurred. You conduct a basic eye examination and find the following: visual acuity in the left eye is 20/60 and does not improve with a pinhole lens; the swinging-flashlight test discloses a left relative afferent pupillary defect; a confrontation visual field test suggests a temporal defect in the left eye only; and ophthalmoscopy reveals mild pallor of the left optic disc. What is the differential diagnosis? Is additional testing required at this time, or should the patient merely be observed further?

   Answer: The history of slowly progressive visual loss and the presence of a relative afferent pupillary defect are evidence of a left optic nerve lesion. Optic neuritis is a possibility, but it usually produces sudden onset of visual loss, with recovery after a few weeks or months. The history and the findings are strongly suggestive of a tumor compressing the left optic nerve. Detailed visual field testing will probably reveal a major field defect in the left eye and a normal field in the right eye. This localizes the lesion to the prechiasmal optic nerve, either in the orbit or in the brain. A CT scan or MRI with and without gadolinium would be the test to order next, with the expectation that it will show a meningioma or another kind of mass compressing the optic nerve.

4. A patient cannot see in the temporal visual field in either eye. Which one of the following findings is *most* likely to be associated with this defect?
   a. tilted optic discs
   b. pituitary tumor
   c. neurofibromatosis
   d. optic nerve toxicity
   e. infarction

   Answer: b. The fact that the field loss respects the vertical meridian in each eye localizes the pathology to the optic chiasm. Pituitary tumor is the most common cause of a chiasmal syndrome. Tilted optic discs can produce temporal field loss, but the defects would extend only up to the blind spot and not to the vertical meridian. Neurofibromatosis can be associated with chiasmal glioma, but pituitary tumor is a more common association. This is not the picture of optic nerve toxicity, which is typically characterized by bilateral central scotomas with intact peripheral fields. Infarction rarely occurs in the chiasm.

5. A 64-year-old woman reports progressive onset of ptosis and diplopia over an 8-month period. On examination, the left eye is normal but the right eye reveals 4 mm of ptosis, limitation of eye movement in all directions, a 4-mm pupil that does not react to light or dilate in darkness, and loss of corneal sensation. Which of the following is the *most* likely diagnosis?
   a. myasthenia gravis
   b. Graves' ophthalmopathy
   c. intracavernous meningioma
   d. aneurysm of the posterior communicating artery
   e. glioma of the right midbrain

   Answer: c. The patient's findings can best be explained by involvement of the third, sixth, fifth, and sympathetic nerves. Fourth-nerve involvement cannot be determined from the description. A middilated pupil that does not react to light or dilate in darkness usually indicates impairment of both the parasympathetic and the sympathetic innervation of the pupil. This finding as well as the other findings can best be explained by a lesion in the cavernous sinus. Meningioma and internal carotid artery aneurysm are the most common causes, particularly with a history of slow progression. Myasthenia gravis and Graves' ophthalmopathy would not produce the pupillary or sensory findings noted in this patient. An aneurysm of the posterior communicating artery could produce a third-nerve palsy but would not be expected to produce the other findings. A midbrain lesion typically produces bilateral ptosis, if any, and could not explain the sensory findings.

Annotated Resources

Glaser JS: *Neuro-ophthalmology*. 2nd ed. Philadelphia: JB Lippincott Co; 1990. This is an excellent, readable reference in neuro-ophthalmology, concise yet thorough. A new edition is due late in 1998.

Keltner JL, Wand M, Van Newkirk MR: *Techniques for the Basic Ocular Examination*. San Francisco: American Academy of Ophthalmology; 1989. This videotape covers visual acuity testing, ocular motility testing, confrontation field testing, glaucoma screening, and ophthalmoscopy.

Miller NR, Newman N: *Walsh & Hoyt's Clinical Neuro-Ophthalmology*. 5th ed. Baltimore: Williams & Wilkins; 1997. This multivolume set is the complete reference for clinical neuro-ophthalmology—the encyclopedia on the subject. Most importantly, it contains a thorough review of the literature.

Spalton DJ, Hitchins RA, Hunter PA: *Atlas of Clinical Ophthalmology*. St Louis: Mosby-Year Book; 1994. The neuro-ophthalmology section in this atlas is very good.

Trobe JD: *The Physician's Guide to Eye Care*. San Francisco: American Academy of Ophthalmology; 1993. A brief but comprehensive resource covering the principal clinical ophthalmic problems that nonophthalmologist physicians are likely to encounter, organized for practical use by practitioners.

Chapter 8

Ocular Manifestations of Systemic Disease

Objectives

As a primary care physician, you should be aware that most systemic diseases have ocular signs and symptoms and that serious ocular sequelae may result from these diseases. You should become familiar with the important features of several of these conditions, including diabetes mellitus, sickle cell anemia, hypertension, thyroid disease, sarcoidosis and inflammatory conditions, malignancy, acquired immunodeficiency syndrome, syphilis, and other systemic infections.

To achieve these objectives, you should learn

- To perform a thorough eye examination (see Chapter 1)
- To recognize the characteristic features, especially the ophthalmoscopic features, of these diseases
- To determine when it is appropriate to refer a patient to an ophthalmologist for consultation or treatment

Relevance

Recognition of the ocular signs, symptoms, and complications of many systemic diseases is vitally important for good medical practice. Diabetes mellitus affects nearly 16 million Americans and is the leading cause of new cases of blindness in working-age Americans. Treatment of diabetic retinopathy is directed toward the prevention of visual loss. Several national clinical trials sponsored by the National Eye Institute have demonstrated that with appropriate referral and treatment the incidence of severe visual loss can be reduced by at least 90%. Acquired immunodeficiency syndrome is a disease of epidemic proportions. More than 75% of AIDS patients have ocular involvement of some kind (from asymptomatic retinal infarctions to vision-threatening cytomegalovirus retinitis). Because ocular findings may reflect disease progression, regular ophthalmologic examination can be beneficial in initiating or modifying treatment in a timely fashion.

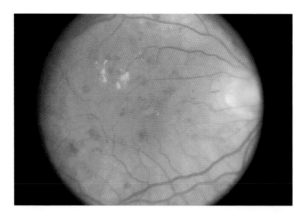

Slide 65
Nonproliferative diabetic retinopathy. Dot-and-blot hemorrhages and exudates are shown scattered throughout the posterior pole. Microaneurysms (pin-point dots) are difficult to see without high magnification.

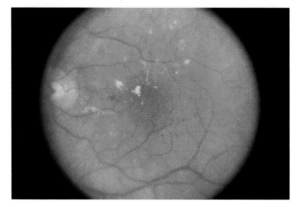

Slide 66   Exudates in nonproliferative diabetic retinopathy. Clusters of hard, yellowish exudates are prominent in the superior aspect of the macula. The exudates extend to the fovea, threatening the central vision.

Diabetes Mellitus

Although diabetes may have a number of ocular effects (eg, cataracts, changes in refractive status), the most important ocular complication is retinopathy.

The longer a person suffers from diabetes, the greater the likelihood of developing diabetic retinopathy. About 5 years after diagnosis, 23% of patients with insulin-dependent diabetes mellitus (IDDM, Type I) have diabetic retinopathy, and after 15 years, 80% have retinopathy. Diabetic patients who have non–insulin-dependent diabetes mellitus (NIDDM, Type II) have a similar but slightly lower incidence of retinopathy. Because patients with Type II diabetes may not be diagnosed until years after onset of their disease, many patients already have significant retinopathy at the time of diagnosis.

The initial stage of the ocular disease is called *nonproliferative diabetic retinopathy* (NPDR). Capillaries develop leaks and later become occluded. The retinal findings of mild and moderate NPDR include microaneurysms, dot-and-blot hemorrhages, hard exudates, and macular edema (Slides 65 and 66). Patients experience visual loss only if there is clinically significant macular edema (CSME), which is present in from 5% to 15% of diabetic

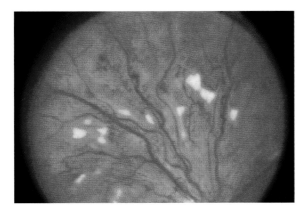

Slide 67   Cotton-wool spots in nonproliferative diabetic retinopathy. Microinfarctions of the nerve fiber layer produce the lesions shown. Cotton-wool spots are opaque and white, have feathery edges, and obscure the underlying blood vessels. Venous beading and telangiectasia of the retinal vasculature are shown.

patients, depending on the type and duration of the disease. CSME is the most common cause of mild to moderate visual loss from diabetic retinopathy.

In time, some patients progress to severe NPDR, which heralds the onset of the most serious form of retinopathy, the proliferative stage. Severe NPDR is marked by increased vascular tortuosity and hemorrhagic activity, venous beading, and widespread intraretinal microvascular abnormalities; it may also include many microinfarctions of the nerve fiber layer, or cotton-wool spots (Slide 67). Of patients diagnosed with severe NPDR, 40% will develop proliferative diabetic retinopathy within 1 year.

Proliferative diabetic retinopathy (PDR) is responsible for most of the profound visual loss from diabetes. As a response to continued retinal ischemia, new blood vessels (neovascularization) form in the area of the optic disc or elsewhere on the retinal surface (Slides 68 and 69). Neovascularization can occur elsewhere in the eye; for example, on the surface of the iris (rubeosis iridis), causing severe glaucoma.

If an eye with proliferative retinopathy is not treated, these fragile new vessels will bleed into the vitreous. Fibrous tissue that accompanies the new vessels will contract and cause a traction retinal detachment. Once these severe complications (massive vitreous hemorrhage or traction retinal detachment) have occurred, laser surgery is unlikely to be effective and a vitrectomy may be necessary in the attempt to restore some vision.

PDR and CSME often remain asymptomatic well beyond the optimal stage for treatment. All patients with diabetes should be referred to an ophthalmologist for examination and followup. Some patients with macular edema will require laser surgery (focal treatment) to areas of leaking blood vessels. This treatment has been demonstrated to reduce visual loss by approximately 50%. All patients with nonproliferative and proliferative retinopathy require frequent ophthalmoscopic examinations, and some require specialized examination techniques such as fluorescein angiography to document the extent of the vascular abnormalities and to guide therapy. Detection of treatable macular edema and proliferative retinopathy requires stereoscopic biomicroscopy and indirect opthalmoscopy through dilated pupils. Examination with the hand-held direct ophthalmoscope is not sufficient to rule out significant, treatable diabetic retinopathy.

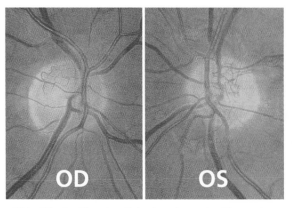

Slide 68   Proliferative diabetic retinopathy. These photographs are from the same patient. The right optic nerve has two new vessels over the superior aspect of the optic nerve. The left optic nerve has more advanced neovascularization. To prevent progression of the neovascularization and possible vitreous hemorrhage, panretinal photocoagulation is required.

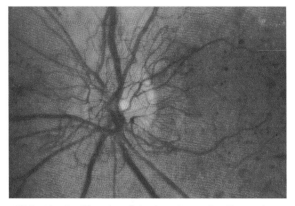

Slide 69   Proliferative diabetic retinopathy. Shown here is more advanced neovascularization of the optic nerve. These new vessels proliferate and extend into the vitreous.

In treating proliferative retinopathy, the ophthalmologist scatters 1000 to 2000 laser burns over the entire surface of the retina except the macula and the papillomacular bundle (Slide 70). This treatment is based on the concept that a reduction of the metabolic oxygen requirement of the retina promotes regression of the neovascular tissue. Appropriately timed effective panretinal laser photocoagulation surgery can reduce the incidence of severe visual loss by at least 50% and as much as 90%. Many patients require frequent treatments when the disease is actively progressing.

All persons with diabetes should be examined at the time of diagnosis and thereafter annually by an ophthalmologist. More frequent examinations are required for patients who have poor glycemic control, hypertension, proteinuria, or anemia, as they are at higher risk for more rapid progression of their retinopathy. Patients who have already been treated with laser

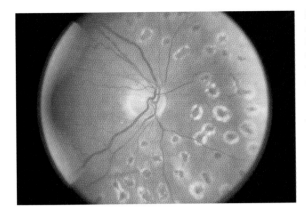

Slide 70   Panretinal argon laser photocoagulation. Shown here are old argon laser burns in the posterior pole of a diabetic patient with proliferative retinopathy. Initially the burns are white, but with time they develop variable pigmentation from chorioretinal scarring.

surgery or vitrectomy should adhere to a followup schedule determined by their ophthalmologist. It is not unusual to require additional treatment.

Pregnant patients with Type I diabetes should be examined by an ophthalmologist during the first trimester and every 3 months thereafter until completion of the pregnancy. Ideally, women who are planning a pregnancy should have a baseline ophthalmologic examination before conception, as pregnancy can severely exacerbate diabetic retinopathy.

The Diabetes Control and Complications Trial (DCCT) showed that intensive glycemic control is associated with a reduced risk of newly diagnosed retinopathy and reduced progression of existing retinopathy in people with insulin-dependent diabetes mellitus (IDDM). Furthermore, the DCCT showed that intensive glycemic control (compared to conventional treatment) was associated with reduction in progression to severe nonproliferative and proliferative retinopathy, incidence of macular edema, and need for panretinal and focal photocoagulation. Advanced diabetic retinopathy is associated with cardiovascular disease risk factors. Patients with proliferative diabetic retinopathy are also at increased risk of heart attack, stroke, diabetic nephropathy, amputation, and death. The results of the DCCT showed that the lowering of blood glucose reduces not only ocular complications but also other end-organ complications, including nephropathy, neuropathy, and cardiovascular disease. It is important that all patients with Type I and most patients with Type II diabetes be educated about the importance of determining and maintaining glycosylated hemoglobin levels to improve glycemic control.

Sickle Cell Anemia

Patients with SC and S Thal disease are more likely to have ocular involvement due to sickle cell than patients with SS disease. Intravascular sickling, hemolysis, hemostasis, and then thrombosis lead to arteriolar occlusion followed by capillary nonperfusion. As with diabetes, inadequate perfusion of the retina can stimulate neovascularization, which can lead to vitreous hemorrhage and retinal detachment. Appropriately timed laser surgery can prevent many vision-threatening complications in these patients.

Hypertension

To understand the effects of systemic hypertension on the retinal vasculature, it is helpful to divide hypertensive retinopathy into two classifications: changes due to arteriolar sclerosis, and changes due to elevated blood pressure.

Arteriolar Sclerosis

Although aging causes thickening and sclerosis of the arterioles, prolonged systemic hypertension (usually, diastolic pressure greater than 100 mm Hg) accelerates this process. Thickening of the walls of the retinal arterioles results in characteristic ophthalmoscopic features of retinal arteriolar sclerosis: changes in the light reflex of the arteriole, and changes in arteriovenous (AV) crossing. The amount of arteriolar sclerosis depends on the duration and severity of the hypertension and may reflect the condition of the arterioles elsewhere in the body.

In a normal eye, the retinal arterioles are transparent tubes with blood visible by ophthalmoscopy; a light streak is reflected from the convex wall of the arteriole. As arteriolar sclerosis causes thickening and fibrosis of the vessel wall, the central light reflex increases in width (Slide 71). After sclerosis progresses, the light reflex occupies most of the width of the vessels; at this point, the vessels are called *copper-wire arterioles*. As fibrosis continues, the light reflex is obscured totally and the arterioles appear whitish and are referred to as *silver-wire arterioles*.

Because the arterioles and veins share a common sheath within the retinal tissue at crossing sites, arteriovenous crossing changes can be seen (Slide 72). There may be zones of concealment where the vein is hidden in the region that underlies the artery. The concealment appears as narrowing (so-called nicking) of the vein as it fades on either side of the arteriole.

The vein may be elevated or depressed by the arteriole and, in more severe cases, may undergo an abrupt right-angle change in course just as it reaches the arteriole (see Slide 72). Alterations in the caliber of the vein may occur because of compression and constriction at the A/V crossing, resulting in dilation of the distal portion of the vein. All of these A/V crossing

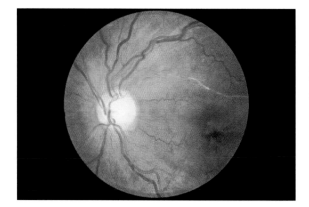

Slide 71 Hypertensive retinopathy. A single retinal vessel with areas of copper-wiring and silver-wiring is visible in this patient with long-standing hypertension.

changes are most significant when found at or beyond the second bifurcation of the arteriole, which is about 1 disc diameter distal to the optic nerve head. A/V nicking can lead to branch retinal vein occlusions, which can decrease central visual acuity and require laser treatment in certain cases.

Elevated Blood Pressure

A moderate acute rise in blood pressure results in constriction of the arterioles. A severe acute rise in blood pressure (usually, diastolic pressure greater than 120 mm Hg) causes fibrinoid necrosis of the vessel wall, resulting in exudates, cotton-wool spots, flame-shaped hemorrhages, and sometimes whitish swelling and edema of large portions of the retina. In the most severe form of hypertensive retinopathy, malignant hypertension (Slide 73), the optic disc swelling that occurs resembles the swelling seen in papilledema.

Diagnostic Concerns

The changes due to acute hypertension are best seen (and sometimes only seen) in previously normal arterioles; that is, in those not affected by arteriolar sclerosis, because the thickening and fibrosis of the vessel walls protect

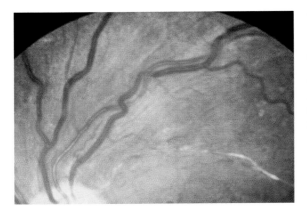

Slide 72   Arteriovenous crossing changes. In this magnified view of Slide 71, an abrupt right-angle change of a vein is visible at the first AV crossing, and nicking of the vein is seen at the second AV crossing.

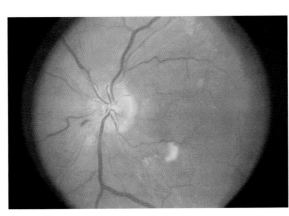

Slide 73   Malignant hypertension. This figure demonstrates the ocular findings associated with severe hypertension: optic nerve swelling, extreme arterial constriction, hemorrhages, early exudates, and cotton-wool spots. Untreated, the optic nerve swelling may progress to resemble papilledema.

against fibrinoid necrosis. For instance, arteriolar sclerosis might mask hypertensive changes in a young patient with a pheochromocytoma or in a pregnant woman with toxemia.

It may be difficult to differentiate chronic hypertensive vascular changes (ie, arteriolar sclerosis) from normal involutional (ie, age-related) changes. In order of importance, the most sensitive ophthalmoscopic indicators of hypertension are attenuation of the retinal arterioles, focal narrowing, and A/V crossing changes.

Management

The primary goal in managing systemic hypertension is adequate control of the blood pressure to preserve the integrity of the cerebral, cardiac, and renal circulations. A sudden, severe increase in blood pressure also can compromise the retinal and choroidal circulations, resulting in loss of vision or visual field. Under these circumstances, the blood pressure should be lowered in a controlled fashion because a sudden drop in tissue perfusion could result in optic nerve infarction and permanent loss of vision.

Thyroid Disease

Graves' disease is an example of an important autoimmune disease that may have ocular manifestations. A common clinical feature of thyroid eye disease is retraction of the upper and lower eyelid, with upper-lid lag on downgaze. Thyroid eye disease is also the most common cause of unilateral or bilateral protrusion of the globes, or exophthalmos, in adults. Exophthalmos (proptosis) in combination with retraction of the eyelids may produce an appearance referred to as *thyroid stare* (Slide 74).

Both eyelid retraction and exophthalmos may result in corneal exposure and drying, causing the patient to complain of a foreign-body sensation and tearing. These bothersome symptoms usually can be relieved by the frequent instillation of over-the-counter artificial-tear preparations and the application of lubricating eye ointment at night. The eyelid edema and

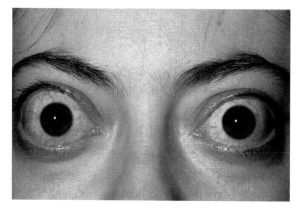

Slide 74 Thyroid stare. The staring appearance of this patient is due to forward protrusion of the eyes and retraction of the eyelids, exposing white sclera above and below the limbus.

conjunctival vascular congestion that sometimes accompany thyroid eye disease usually do not require therapy. Proptosis may be surgically treated if severe and persistent.

Thyroid eye disease may cause other serious complications requiring an ophthalmologist's care. Diplopia due to extraocular muscle involvement is common and may require strabismus surgery. Compression of the optic nerve within the orbit can cause loss of vision, necessitating surgery to decompress the orbit or irradiation to reduce the inflammatory swelling of the muscles.

Sarcoidosis and Inflammatory Conditions

Sarcoidosis is a chronic disease of uncertain derivation that affects several organ systems, including the eye. Ocular manifestations are characterized histologically by the presence of focal noncaseating granulomas. Sarcoidosis is most common in African-American women aged 20 to 40. Laboratory findings include increased serum calcium (12% of patients), lack of energy (50% of patients), elevated angiotensin-converting enzyme (75% of patients), and abnormal results on chest x-ray (80% of patients). Important histopathologic information also can be obtained from ocular tissues. The easiest tissue from which to obtain a biopsy specimen is the conjunctiva, but tissue from the lacrimal gland may be obtained as it is also a frequent locus of granulomatous infiltration. Both of these biopsy procedures can be performed under local anesthesia; these areas should be considered before performing potentially more complicated mediastinal or transbronchial biopsies of lymph nodes.

Because ocular involvement from sarcoidosis may be asymptomatic, all patients suspected of sarcoidosis should have a complete ophthalmic evaluation. Sarcoidosis may cause anterior or posterior uveitis. Anterior uveitis is inflammation of the iris and ciliary body (Slide 75); posterior uveitis is inflammation of the choroid. Early initiation of topical or systemic corticosteroids is effective and may prevent complications, such as

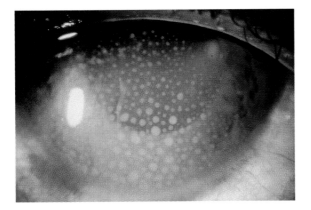

Slide 75 Anterior uveitis. Inflammatory cells collect on the inner surface of the cornea, producing opacities called keratic precipitates.

glaucoma, cataract, and adhesions of the iris to the lens. Involvement of the retina is usually associated with posterior uveitis and may include perivasculitis, hemorrhages, and neovascularization of the peripheral retina. Involvement of the central nervous system is twice as common when the fundus is involved, increasing from 10% or 15% to between 20% and 30%. Ophthalmic manifestations of neurosarcoidosis include optic neuropathy, oculomotor abnormalities (including sixth-nerve palsy), and, rarely, chiasmal and retrochiasmal visual field loss.

Dry eye caused by reduced tear production may be seen in sarcoidosis because of lacrimal gland infiltration, but it also occurs in a variety of rheumatologic conditions. The most common are systemic lupus erythematosus and rheumatoid arthritis. Dry eye also is common in a mild form in healthy individuals over age 40. Symptoms include a sensation of burning or grittiness of the eyes, especially late in the day. Accumulation of mucus on the eyelids also occurs in affected patients upon awakening. Many patients complain of tearing, presumably after the eye becomes dry enough to stimulate reflex tearing. Treatment includes the application of artificial tears and occasionally lubricating ointment at night. In the vast majority of patients, the condition is annoying, but rarely leads to serious ocular problems. Occasional patients with advanced rheumatoid arthritis develop severe drying, have corneal damage, and are at greater risk for corneal infection.

Juvenile rheumatoid arthritis is an important childhood systemic condition with ocular manifestations. About 10% of all juvenile rheumatoid arthritis patients have iritis, but the inflammation is more common with the pauciarticular form of the disease (20% to 30% of patients) and much less common in the polyarticular form. Patients who have juvenile rheumatoid arthritis, especially the pauciarticular form, require visits to the ophthalmologist every 3 months because the iritis is commonly asymptomatic. If inflammation is not recognized, extensive ocular complications arise, including cataract, glaucoma, and calcification of the cornea. Iritis is also a common complication of ankylosing spondylitis (10% to 15% of affected patients), Reiter's syndrome, and Behçet's disease.

Malignancy

Cancer originating within the eye or ocular adnexa is rare. More often, the eye is affected secondarily by cancer or by the various forms of cancer therapy. Ocular and orbital metastases are found in up to 5% of cancer patients at autopsy, most often from the breast or the lung. Usually, the tumors infiltrate the choroid, but the optic nerve as well as the extraocular muscles also may be affected. Systemic lymphoma affects the eye in about 3% of patients by infiltrating the conjunctiva or the orbit and causing proptosis or limitation of extraocular movement. In children, leukemic infiltration of ocular tissues can occur. More than 75% of leukemia patients seen at autopsy have ocular adnexal metastases. Commonly, patients with leukemia develop superficial retinal, preretinal, or subconjunctival hemorrhages as a result of thrombocytopenia or the effects of transfusion on normal clotting. Cancer may have remote effects on the eye, including autonomic dysfunction of the pupils as well as a rare but devastating retinal degeneration that has a presumed autoimmune pathogenesis.

Radiation of tumors in the vicinity of the eye may lead to the development of cataract. The lens is susceptible to doses of radiation in the range of 2000 rads. Radiation damage causes a delayed retinal vasculopathy and optic neuropathy. A variety of cancer chemotherapeutic agents have secondary ocular effects. Superficial keratitis may be caused by cytosine arabinoside, optic neuropathy may occur with vincristine injections, and retinal artery occlusion may be caused by carotid artery injection of BCNU (carmustine). Mucosal damage from graft-vs-host disease may involve the conjunctiva, leading to dryness and corneal decompensation with subsequent infection.

Acquired Immunodeficiency Syndrome

Acquired immunodeficiency syndrome (AIDS) is a severe disorder in which depression of the immune system results in the development of multiple opportunistic infections and malignancies. Ophthalmic examination may confirm the diagnosis. Common ophthalmic manifestations are cotton-wool spots (AIDS retinopathy), cytomegalovirus retinitis, and Kaposi's sarcoma affecting the eyelids. The less common complications include herpes zoster (shingles), herpes simplex keratitis, conjunctival microangiopathy, luetic and toxoplasmic uveitis and retinitis, and visual field defects or oculomotor dysfunction resulting from central nervous system involvement.

Retinal cotton-wool spots (Slide 76) are due to the focal occlusions of retinal capillaries that result in accumulation of axoplasm in the region of the retinal nerve fiber layer. In AIDS, the occlusions are thought to be due to microthrombi from antigen-antibody complexes and fibrin. These are frequently the sole ocular finding in patients with AIDS (more than 50%). Cotton-wool spots and hemorrhages with white centers are found in

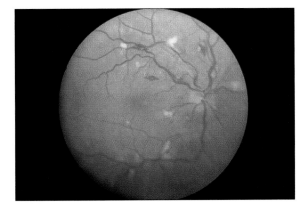

Slide 76 Cotton-wool spots in AIDS. Scattered cotton-wool spots, as well as some hemorrhages, are depicted in this retina of a patient with AIDS.

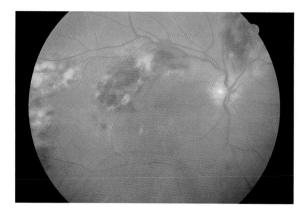

Slide 77
Cytomegalovirus retinitis in AIDS. The multicentric retinitis is characterized by discrete, fluffy, white retinal necrosis, with retinal hemorrhages and vasculitis. There is a sharp, distinct border between the diseased retina and the normal retina.

patients with a variety of other infectious conditions, including subacute bacterial endocarditis and systemic candidiasis.

Cytomegalovirus (CMV) retinitis (Slide 77) is the leading cause of visual loss in patients with AIDS, occurring in more than 25% of patients. The distinctive ophthalmoscopic appearance of CMV retinitis is characterized by hemorrhagic necrosis of the retina. Areas of involved retina have distinct borders and abruptly abut areas of normal retina. The disease progresses over weeks to months and results in total atrophy of the affected retina. Most patients who develop CMV retinitis have a poor prognosis for survival.

Kaposi's sarcoma, characterized by multiple vascular skin malignancies, may involve the conjunctiva of either the lid or the globe. Unless suspected, this sarcoma may be misdiagnosed as a subconjunctival hemorrhage or a hemangioma.

Until recently, therapeutic intervention has been aimed at halting progression of the opportunistic infection. However, with the advent of protease inhibitors, some patients have shown resolution of their opportunistic infection.

Any patient with a diagnosis of HIV should be referred to an ophthalmologist for a complete ophthalmologic examination. Detailed discussion of therapeutic intervention is beyond the scope of this book. However, when such intervention is indicated, many variables must be considered, and it is important that good communication be established among the patient's other treating physicians and that therapy be determined based on a team approach.

Syphilis

Intraocular inflammation due to syphilis can be cured, even in patients with AIDS. Delay in diagnosis of syphilitic chorioretinitis can lead to permanent visual loss that might have been avoided with early treatment.

Acute interstitial keratitis with keratouveitis occurs in patients with congenital syphilis between the ages of 5 and 25 years. It is bilateral in congenital disease and unilateral if acquired. It is believed to be an allergic

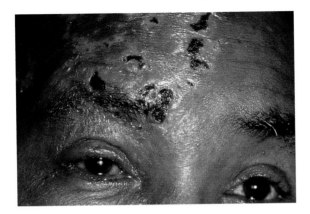

Slide 78 Herpes zoster ophthalmicus. Crusting lesions (no longer vesicles) are present in the distribution of the ophthalmic division of the fifth cranial nerve. The conjunctiva is red and the lids are swollen, indicating ocular involvement by herpes zoster. (Fluorescein has been instilled.)

response to *Treponema pallidum* in the cornea. Symptoms and signs include intense pain and photophobia, and a diffusely opaque cornea with vision reduced, even to light perception. Blood vessels invade the cornea, and when they meet in the center of the cornea after several months, the inflammation subsides and the cornea partially clears. Late stages show deep ghost (nonperfused) stromal vessels and opacities. Any patient with syphilitic uveitis should have a spinal fluid examination.

Ocular involvement in secondary syphilis may feature pain, redness, or photophobia, or blurred vision and floating spots. The patient may present with iritis or choroiditis. There may be exudates around the disc and along the retinal arterioles in secondary syphilis. Arteritis and periarteritis may occur.

In latent syphilis, the presenting ocular complaint is usually blurred vision. The presence of chorioretinitis usually indicates cerebrospinal fluid involvement or neurosyphilis. Diffuse neuroretinitis with papillitis and periarterial sheathing may also occur.

Other Systemic Infections

In addition to AIDS, other systemic infections may affect the eye. The most common are candidiasis and herpes zoster. The typical *Candida* lesion is a fluffy, white-yellow, superficial retinal infiltrate that may lead to the rapid development of overlying vitreous haze and eventual vitritis. Rarely, inflammation of the anterior chamber occurs. The presence of ocular candidiasis is a specific indication for systemic therapy with amphotericin B.

Herpes zoster ophthalmicus (Slide 78), from varicella zoster involving the ophthalmic division of the fifth cranial nerve, may result in ocular manifestations, especially when vesicles appear on the tip of the nose from extension along the nasociliary branch. Corneal infiltration with the virus may lead to disruption of the epithelium, best seen as fluorescein dye staining of the cornea. However, the epithelium usually heals spontaneously and rapidly. The most important ocular side effect of herpes zoster is anterior uveitis, which can be confirmed by slit-lamp examination. The combination of anterior uveitis and keratitis, especially with loss of normal corneal sensation, is a serious vision-threatening effect. Affected patients should be referred to an ophthalmologist immediately for assistance in diagnosis and treatment. Rare ocular complications of herpes zoster include optic neuritis and oculomotor nerve involvement with subsequent diplopia.

Points to Remember

1. To recognize many ocular manifestations of systemic disease, the primary care physician must perform a thorough fundus examination, preferably through dilated pupils.
2. Early diagnosis of diabetic retinopathy is crucial to the ultimate success of treatment, which is effective for both nonproliferative and proliferative stages of the disease when patients are referred in a timely fashion.
3. Any patient with an autoimmune disease or systemic infection who presents with a red eye, decreased vision, photophobia, or floaters should be referred to an ophthalmologist for a slit-lamp examination to look for subtle but vision-threatening intraocular inflammation.

Sample Problems

1. An adult patient with a 10-year history of non–insulin-dependent diabetes comes to your office for the first time, having recently moved from another state. She tells you that she has never seen an ophthalmologist nor had a dilated ophthalmoscopic examination. Her visual acuity is normal, but on dilated fundus examination, you find neovascularization of the optic disc. How do you manage this patient?

   Answer: Although this patient's visual acuity is normal, neovascularization of the optic disc is diagnostic of proliferative diabetic retinopathy, which places this patient at high risk for developing marked visual loss. She should be referred immediately to an ophthalmologist for examination and treatment. Panretinal laser photocoagulation surgery can be initiated to reverse the course of the neovascularization and reduce the risk of serious visual loss.

2. A 45-year-old man comes to your office complaining of headaches and nosebleeds. His blood pressure is 180/120 mm Hg. On dilated fundus examination, you find numerous exudates, flame-shaped hemorrhages, cotton-wool spots, and severe attenuation of the arterioles. You do not find AV crossing changes, and the arteriolar light reflex is normal. What information does your ophthalmoscopic examination provide about the chronicity of the patient's systemic hypertension?

   Answer: Flame-shaped hemorrhages and cotton-wool spots are ophthalmoscopic changes indicative of acute, severe hypertension. When these features occur in the absence of arteriolar sclerotic changes (ie, AV crossing phenomenon), the hypertension is most likely of recent onset.

In such cases, hypertension may be associated with renal insufficiency, encephalopathy, and impairment of cardiac function. Controlled reduction of blood pressure should be initiated immediately.

3. A previously healthy 40-year-old woman presents with bilateral proptosis and lid retraction, but she denies any pain. The most likely diagnosis is
   a. metastatic tumor to orbit
   b. orbital cellulitis
   c. orbital pseudotumor
   d. thyroid eye disease
   e. carotid artery-cavernous sinus fistula

   Answer: d. Thyroid eye disease is the most common cause of unilateral or bilateral proptosis in adults. Thyroid eye disease can be present with normal thyroid function. Orbital pseudotumor usually causes pain, whereas thyroid eye disease does not. Orbital cellulitis usually presents with swollen, tender, erythematous lids, malaise, and elevated white blood cell count. Carotid cavernous sinus fistula causing proptosis is more common following trauma and is not associated with lid retraction, and often a bruit can be auscultated with the stethoscope over the orbit. Metastatic tumor of the orbit would not likely be bilateral with a negative past medical history.

Annotated Resources

Benson WE, Brown GC, Tasman W: *Diabetes and Its Ocular Complications.* Philadelphia: WB Saunders Co; 1988. A thorough discussion of the many ocular complications of diabetes.

Diabetes Control and Complications Trial Research Group. The effect of intensive treatment of diabetes on the development and progression of long-term complications in insulin-dependent diabetes mellitus. *N Engl J Med* 1993;329:977–986. Intensive therapy effectively delays the onset and slows the progression of diabetic retinopathy, nephropathy, and neuropathy in patients with insulin-dependent diabetes mellitus.

Diabetic Retinopathy Study Research Group: Photocoagulation treatment of proliferative diabetic retinopathy: the second report of diabetic retinopathy study findings. *Ophthalmology* 1978;85:82–106. A report of the findings in this classic prospective, randomized, multicenter study on diabetic retinopathy.

DRSR Group, ETDRSR Group: *Management of Diabetic Retinopathy for the Primary Care Physician.* San Francisco: American Academy of Ophthalmology; 1990. This videotape helps the primary care physician identify and distinguish between the various stages of diabetic retinopathy. It covers the associated risks of each stage, the essentials of followup and treatment, a brief description of the pathophysiology, and the importance of timely referral.

Duane TD, Osher RH, Green WR: White-centered hemorrhages: their significance. *Ophthalmology* 1980;87:66–69. A good review of the causes and pathophysiology of Roth's spots.

Ferry AP, Font RL: Carcinoma metastatic to the eye and orbit, I: a clinical pathologic study of 227 cases. *Arch Ophthalmol* 1974;92:276–286. The classic article on the subject.

Iwata K, Namba K, Sobue K, et al: Ocular sarcoidosis: evaluation of intraocular findings. *Ann NY Acad Sci* 1976;278:445–454. An overview of ocular sarcoidosis with incidences of each occurrence.

Kanski JJ: Juvenile arthritis and uveitis. *Surv Ophthalmol* 1990;34:253–267. A major review of the subject with many references.

Palestine AG, Rodrigues MM, Macher AM, et al: Ophthalmic involvement in acquired immunodeficiency syndrome. *Ophthalmology* 1984; 91:1092–1099. One of the best summaries of the ophthalmic changes associated with the acquired immunodeficiency syndrome.

Parke DW, Jones DB, Genry OO: Endogenic endophthalmitis among patients with candidemia. *Ophthalmology* 1982;89:789–794. A useful study of hospitalized immunocompromised patients who needed ophthalmic consultation.

Results from the early treatment of diabetic retinopathy study. *Ophthalmology* 1991;98(suppl):739–840. A comprehensive review of the current approach to background diabetic retinopathy.

Trobe JD: *The Physician's Guide to Eye Care*. San Francisco: American Academy of Ophthalmology; 1993. A brief but comprehensive resource covering the principal clinical ophthalmic problems that nonophthalmologist physicians are likely to encounter, organized for practical use by practitioners.

Van Dyk HJL: Orbital Graves' disease: a modification of the "NO SPECS" classification. *Ophthalmology* 1981;88:479–483. A clear discussion of the progression of this common disease.

Walsh JB: Hypertensive retinopathy: description, classification and prognosis. *Ophthalmology* 1982;89:1127–1132. A good review of hypertensive effects on the eye with simplification of various classifications.

Chapter 9

Drugs and the Eye

Objectives

As a primary care physician, you should be able to use pharmacologic agents to facilitate an eye examination, including staining the corneal surface with fluorescein, anesthetizing the cornea with a topical anesthetic, and dilating the pupil with one or more mydriatic drugs. You should be aware of the potential ocular complications of the eyedrops and systemic drugs that you prescribe and be able to recognize these ocular complications when they occur. In addition, you should be cognizant of the systemic effects of the topical ophthalmic drugs that an ophthalmologist might prescribe for your patients.

To achieve these objectives, you should learn

■ The technique of applying drugs to the conjunctival sac
■ The ocular effects and complications of common topical ocular drugs used for diagnosis and therapy, including anesthetics, mydriatics, and corticosteroids
■ The systemic side effects of glaucoma medications: beta-adrenergic blockers, cholinergic stimulators, adrenergic drugs, prostaglandin analogs, and carbonic anhydrase inhibitors
■ The ocular side effects of systemically administered corticosteroids, the chloroquines, digitalis, amiodarone, diphenylhydantoin, ethambutol, chlorpromazine, and thioridazine

Relevance

You will need to use diagnostic drugs to perform a complete ocular examination, which entails skills that every primary care physician should possess. You must be familiar with the side effects and complications of diagnostic and therapeutic drugs to minimize the potential for problems and to recognize them when they do occur.

Basic Information

Using the proper technique to instill eyedrops ensures maximum patient cooperation and adequate delivery of medication to the eye. To instill topical ocular medications, follow these steps:

1. Wash your hands; wear disposable gloves if desired.
2. Instruct the seated patient to tilt the head back and to look up.
3. Expose the palpebral conjunctiva by gently pulling downward on the skin over the cheekbone (Figure 9.1). Avoid direct pressure on the eyeball.
4. Instill the correct amount of medication into the lower conjunctival fornix. Avoid applying drops directly to the cornea, which is the most sensitive part of the eye, and avoid touching the tip of the applicator to the patient's lids or eye.
5. Instruct the patient to close both eyes gently for a few seconds. Wipe any excess medication from the patient's skin with a tissue.

Topical Ocular Diagnostic Drugs

The drugs discussed in this section are used in executing a basic eye examination and assessing certain ocular complaints commonly encountered by the primary care physician. Before administering any medication, always ask patients if they may be allergic to the agent.

Fluorescein Dye

Sodium fluorescein is a water-soluble, orange-yellow dye that becomes a brilliant green when viewed under cobalt-blue or fluorescent light. The dye, which does not irritate the eye, is extremely helpful in detecting abrasions of the corneal surface because fluorescein stains damaged epithelium (see Slides 5 and 6 in Chapter 1). To instill the dye, a sterile, individually packaged dry fluorescein strip is moistened with a drop of sterile water or saline and then applied to the inferior bulbar conjunctiva. A few blinks spread the now-visible tear film across the cornea. Although no systemic complications accompany the use of topical fluorescein, a local complication is the staining of a soft contact lens because of its porous structure. To avoid discoloration, contact lenses should be removed before the fluorescein is instilled.

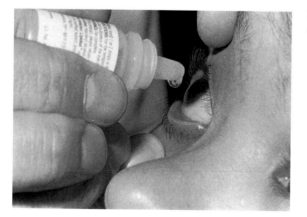

Figure 9.1 Instillation of topical drops.

Anesthetics

Among the topical anesthetics, the most widely used agents are proparacaine hydrochloride 0.5% and tetracaine 0.5%. The instillation of 1 drop of these surface-active compounds renders the corneal epithelium insensate within 15 seconds. Such anesthesia is useful to make surface manipulations painless; for example, to remove a superficial corneal foreign body or perform tonometry. Use of an anesthetic also facilitates the examination of a damaged cornea, which otherwise might be difficult because of the pain. Patients should be instructed not to rub their eyes for at least 10 minutes after receiving topical ocular anesthetics to avoid their inadvertently scratching their corneas.

Topical anesthetics may produce local or systemic allergy, but this is rare. They should never be prescribed for repeated use by patients because they are toxic to the corneal epithelium; they inhibit mitosis and cellular migration and can lead to corneal ulceration and permanent corneal scarring. (See Chapter 4 for a discussion of therapeutic warnings.)

Mydriatics

Mydriatics are drugs that dilate the pupil; dilation may be necessary for ophthalmoscopy. The two classes of mydriatics are cholinergic-blocking (or parasympatholytic) drugs and adrenergic-stimulating (or sympathomimetic) drugs.

Cholinergic-Blocking Drugs

Drugs in this category dilate the pupil by paralyzing the iris sphincter. Several such drugs are in regular use: tropicamide 0.5% or 1%; cyclopentolate hydrochloride 0.5% or 1%, and homatropine hydrobromide 1% or 2%. Atropine sulfate 0.5% or 1% and scopolamine hydrobromide 0.25% or 5% are also available for topical ocular use, but they should never be used just to dilate the pupil for diagnostic purposes because their effects may last 1 to 2 weeks.

Cholinergic-blocking drugs produce not only mydriasis but also cycloplegia, or paralysis of the muscles of the ciliary body. For this reason, these drugs are often referred to as *cycloplegics*. Cycloplegia produces paralysis of accommodation (focusing), so that patients find their near vision may be blurred until the effects of the cycloplegic wear off. Nevertheless, these drugs are widely employed by physicians because they produce excellent mydriasis and the cycloplegic effect facilitates refraction.

Tropicamide is a popular mydriatic with primary care physicians and ophthalmologists alike because of its rapid onset and short duration. Maximum pupillary dilation is attained about 30 minutes after instillation, and the effect diminishes within 4 to 5 hours. Cautions regarding pupillary dilation are discussed in Chapter 1. Systemic side effects of tropicamide are decidedly rare because of its brief duration of action, but they may be serious; they include nausea, vomiting, pallor, and vasomotor collapse. Cyclopentolate produces more complete cycloplegia and is used by ophthalmologists to perform refractions in children.

Adrenergic-Stimulating Drugs

These drugs dilate the pupil by stimulating the pupillary dilator muscle. Only one such drug is in regular use: phenylephrine hydrochloride 2.5%. Just 1 drop applied to the eye dilates the pupil in 30 to 40 minutes, but has no effect on accommodation; thus, phenylephrine is a mydriatic but not a cycloplegic. Because accommodation is not affected, the patient can use near vision after instillation. However, the mydriasis produced is not as great as with tropicamide, and the pupil remains reactive to light. For these reasons, phenylephrine is seldom used alone as a mydriatic.

When maximum mydriasis is required—for example, when the far periphery of the retina must be examined—phenylephrine in combination with tropicamide is ideal because the effects are additive. This combination is often used to dilate the pupil of a brown iris as well, because mydriatics are less effective in dark-eyed individuals than in blue-eyed ones. The 2.5% solution of phenylephrine is much preferred to the 10% solution because the stronger preparation has been associated with acute hypertension and even with myocardial infarction in some patients.

In infants, the combination of cyclopentolate hydrochloride 0.2% and phenylephrine hydrochloride 1.0% (Cyclomydril) is the safest and most effective agent. Hypertension and reduced gastric emptying may occur if stronger agents are used.

Topical Ocular Therapeutic Drugs

The topically applied ocular drugs reviewed in this section are of clinical importance.

Decongestants

This group of drugs is important if only because more than a million bottles of over-the-counter ocular decongestant are purchased each month in the United States. These weak adrenergic-stimulating drugs temporarily whiten the conjunctiva through their vasoconstrictor effect. They are advertised as effective in relieving redness of the eye due to minor eye irritations caused by smoke, dust, smog, wind, glare, swimming, contact lenses, or fatigue.

Naphazoline hydrochloride 0.012%, phenylephrine hydrochloride 0.12%, and tetrahydrozaline hydrochloride 0.05% are the three major drugs in this category. The widespread belief that the use of these compounds is part of good ocular hygiene is a misconception. Red, burning eyes may benefit as much from a cold, wet compress to the closed eyelids as they would from these compounds. Nevertheless, these agents are purchased in high volume.

The most frequent complication of ocular decongestants arises from overuse, with rebound vasodilation of conjunctival vessels. In other words, when used in excess, these preparations can increase rather than decrease redness of the eyes. In rare instances, acute angle-closure glaucoma may be precipitated in susceptible eyes by the use of sympathomimetic drugs because they can dilate the pupil. However, these drugs may be used without harm by patients with chronic open-angle glaucoma because they do not produce a rise in pressure if the filtration angle is open.

Agents for Relief of Allergic Conjunctivitis

Combinations of naphazoline and antazoline or pheniramine drops are available over the counter as remedies for redness and itching associated with seasonal allergic conjunctivitis. These provide decongestant action (see above) as well as antihistamine effects. Prescription medications are also available for management of these symptoms. The mast-cell stabilizers cromolyn and lodoxamide prevent the release of inflammatory mediators and are administered chronically for prevention of allergic symptoms. Levocabastine, an antihistamine, and ketorolac, a nonsteroidal anti-inflammatory agent, are helpful for use as needed for symptomatic relief.

Anti-Inflammatory Agents

Both corticosteroids and nonsteroidal topical preparations are useful in the management of various ocular situations. Topical ocular corticosteroids should never be prescribed by a primary care physician. The serious complications of this class of drugs are discussed in Chapter 4 and include promotion of viral, bacterial, and fungal infections as well as possible development of glaucoma and cataract. Nonsteroidal anti-inflammatory agents do not potentiate these complications. Topical ocular preparations include diclofenac, ketorolac, flurbiprofen, and suprofen. These alone are generally not potent enough to control significant intraocular inflammation, however. They are also used by ophthalmologists for other specific indications, such as ocular itching, macular edema, or prevention of miosis during cataract surgery.

Antibiotics

Topical antibiotics may be used for bacterial infections of the conjunctiva and cornea. The choice of agent is based on the suspected infecting organism. Many commercial agents are available in ophthalmic preparations of drops or ointment.

Topical antibiotics are useful for treating common bacterial conjunctivitis. Useful antibiotics include fluoroquinolones, sulfacetamide, and erythromycin. Neomycin-containing agents, although effective as antibacterials, often cause increased redness and tearing because of topical sensitivity. Antibiotics combined with corticosteroids should be used only under the direction of an ophthalmologist, because the combination may accelerate the progression of a herpes simplex or fungal infection and cause permanent damage.

Systemic Side Effects of Glaucoma Medications

The topically administered glaucoma drugs discussed in this section may have potent systemic side effects. Any drug instilled in the conjunctival cul-de-sac may be absorbed systemically by the conjunctiva, nasopharyngeal mucosa, or gastrointestinal tract (after saliva is swallowed in the nasopharynx). One class of agents, the carbonic anhydrase inhibitors, may also be given orally and may cause side effects as well.

Beta-Adrenergic Blockers

Topical Timolol, Levobunolol, Metapranolol, and Carteolol

Nonselective beta-adrenergic antagonists reduce the formation of aqueous humor by the ciliary body and thereby reduce intraocular pressure. Timolol and its analogs levobunolol, metapranolol, and carteolol are highly effective and widely used. Because the systemic beta-adrenergic effects include bronchospasm, these drugs are contraindicated in patients with asthma or chronic obstructive pulmonary disease. Several deaths have been reported secondary to the pulmonary complications of topically administered timolol. Because of their cardiac effects, topical beta-adrenergic antagonists may precipitate or worsen cardiac failure and must be used with caution if bradycardia or systemic hypotension would adversely affect the patient.

Topical Betaxolol

A cardioselective beta-1-adrenergic antagonist, betaxolol hydrochloride was developed to avoid the pulmonary complications of timolol. Betaxolol may be as effective as nonselective beta-adrenergic antagonists in lowering intraocular pressure. However, pulmonary effects have occasionally been noted, and caution should be used when this drug is employed in patients with excessive impairment of pulmonary function.

Cholinergic-Stimulating Drugs

Topical Pilocarpine

Pilocarpine, available in drop and ointment forms, lowers intraocular pressure by increasing aqueous outflow through the trabecular meshwork. Because of frequent local side effects, including diminished vision due to pupillary constriction and headaches from ciliary muscle spasm, this drop is a less popular glaucoma agent. Systemic side effects are rare, however, as systemic toxicity occurs only at 5 to 10 times the usual ocular dosage. Nevertheless, lacrimation, salivation, perspiration, nausea, vomiting, and diarrhea may occasionally occur, especially with overdosage.

Topical Echothiophate

A long-acting anticholinesterase, echothiophate iodide also mimics stimulation of the parasympathetic nervous system and is, therefore, used clinically to treat glaucoma and occasionally accommodative esotropia. The side effects of echothiophate are identical to those described for pilocarpine but are more common. In addition, because long-term use of this drug inactivates plasma cholinesterase, patients are more susceptible to the effects of succinylcholine and procaine because plasma cholinesterase hydrolyzes those agents. Prolonged apnea and even death have been reported from the use of succinylcholine during anesthesia in patients with low blood cholinesterase secondary to treatment with topical ocular echothiophate.

Alpha-2 Adrenoreceptor Agonists

Topical Brimonidine

Brimonidine tartrate is a relatively selective alpha-2 agonist that lowers intraocular pressure by a presumed dual mechanism of decreased aqueous production and increased uveoscleral (non–trabecular meshwork) aqueous outflow. To date, systemic side effects of this new glaucoma medication have been few but may include oral dryness, headache, and fatigue and drowsiness. Brimonidine should not be given to infants because of the risk of severe hypotension and apnea. In adults it may cause a local allergic reaction.

Topical Apraclonidine

Apraclonidine, a derivative of clonidine, decreases aqueous formation and increases uveoscleral outflow. It is primarily utilized for temporary intraocular pressure control in critical situations or as prophylaxis against pressure spikes after glaucoma laser procedures, but it may also be used chronically to treat glaucoma. Its most concerning systemic side effects include promotion of orthostatic hypotension and vasovagal episodes. Locally it has a fairly high rate of sensitivity reaction and may cause an impressive contact dermatitis of the lids and conjunctiva. Use of topical apraclonidine is associated with mild pupillary dilation, whitening of the conjunctiva, and elevation of the upper eyelid.

Adrenergic-Stimulating Drugs

Topical Epinephrine and Dipivefrin

Epinephrine hydrochloride and dipivefrin, an epinephrine prodrug, are occasionally used in the treatment of glaucoma. Epinephrine in particular may cause cardiac arrhythmia or an increase in systemic blood pressure in some patients due to its adrenergic stimulation.

Prostaglandin Analog

Topical Latanoprost

A relatively new glaucoma medication, latanoprost is a synthetic analog of prostaglandin $F_{2\alpha}$. It increases aqueous outflow through the uveoscleral pathway, a supplemental route through which a small portion of the aqueous drains. No major, concerning systemic toxic effects of this drug have been reported, but it has the peculiar potential to darken iris color in some patients with blue, green, or hazel irides. Latanoprost also has been associated with lengthening and increased fullness of eyelashes in treated eyes. In addition, it may cause swelling of the macula in patients who have had cataract extractions.

Carbonic Anhydrase Inhibitors

Oral Acetazolamide, Methazolamide, and Dichlorphenamide

These aqueous suppressants are the only oral drugs utilized for glaucoma management. Their use, particularly on a chronic basis, is limited by a number of side effects, which include paresthesias, anorexia, gastrointestinal disturbances, headaches, altered taste and smell, sodium and potassium depletion, and a predisposition to form renal calculi, and rarely, bone marrow suppression.

Topical Dorzolamide

Topical dorzolamide lowers intraocular pressure by the same mechanism as oral carbonic anhydrase inhibitors. It has a significantly lower (but still possible) incidence of systemic side effects.

Ocular Side Effects of Systemic Drugs

The drugs covered in this section are systemically administered medications that may have profound ocular or neuro-ocular effects.

Corticosteroids

Corticosteroids or, more properly, adrenocorticosteroids, when given long-term in moderate dosage, produce posterior subcapsular cataracts. Asthmatic individuals, renal-transplant recipients, and patients with rheumatoid arthritis are groups in whom this phenomenon has been commonly observed. Patients with rheumatoid arthritis may develop posterior subcapsular cataracts in the absence of corticosteroid therapy, but the incidence increases with corticosteroid therapy. The use of systemic or inhaled corticosteroids is associated with elevated intraocular pressures (steroid-induced glaucoma) in susceptible individuals.

Chloroquines

Chloroquine phosphate and hydroxychloroquine sulfate, originally used to treat malaria, are now also used to treat rheumatoid arthritis, lupus erythematosus, and other autoimmune disorders. Chloroquines can produce corneal deposits and retinopathy. The corneal deposits are usually asymptomatic, but can produce glare and photophobia. The deposits regress when the drug is discontinued, but the retinopathy is much more serious. This drug-induced retinal damage is insidious, slowly progressive, and usually irreversible. The typical bull's-eye macular lesions do not become visible ophthalmoscopically until serious retinal damage has already occurred. Patients taking high dosages of chloroquine phosphate (eg, more than 250 mg a day) or having long-term treatment (eg, 3 or more years of at least 300 g total dosage) are at greatest risk. Patients using the chloroquines require regular ophthalmologic examinations, with visual acuity, color vision, Amsler grid, visual field, and ophthalmoscopic testing at the minimum.

Digitalis

Intoxication with this widely used cardiovascular drug almost always produces blurred vision or abnormally colored vision (ie, chromatopsia). Classically, normal objects appear yellow with the overdosage of digitalis, but green, red, brown, or blue vision can also occur. White halos may be perceived on dark objects, or objects may seem frosted in appearance. Usually, fatigue and weakness develop concomitantly with digitalis intoxication, but the visual disturbances often dominate the patient's complaints.

Amiodarone

Amiodarone is a cardiac arrhythmia drug that produces whorl-shaped, pigmented deposits in the corneal epithelium. These deposits are dosage-related and reversible if the dosage is decreased or the drug is discontinued entirely. Visual symptoms are rare.

Diphenylhydantoin

Still widely used for the control of seizures, diphenylhydantoin sodium causes dosage-related cerebellar-vestibular effects. Horizontal nystagmus in lateral gaze, vertical nystagmus in upgaze, vertigo, ataxia, and even diplopia occur with mildly elevated blood levels of the drug. More complex forms of nystagmus and even ophthalmoplegia may accompany extremely high blood levels. These effects are reversible if the drug is discontinued.

Ethambutol

Ethambutol is useful in the chemotherapy of tuberculosis. As a side effect, ethambutol produces a dosage-related optic neuropathy. With dosages of 15 mg/kg/day, optic neuropathy occurs in less than 1% of patients, but increases to 5% of patients receiving 25 mg/kg/day and to 15% receiving 50 mg/kg/day. The onset of visual loss may be within 1 month of starting the drug. Recovery usually occurs when the drug is stopped, but may take months; occasionally, visual loss is permanent.

Chlorpromazine

This psychoactive drug produces punctate opacities in the corneal epithelium after long-term use. Occasionally, opacities develop on the lens surface as well. These opacities rarely cause symptoms and are reversible with discontinuation of the drug.

Thioridazine

Thioridazine, commonly used to treat patients with psychoses, produces a pigmentary retinopathy after high dosage, usually at least 1000 mg/day. The current recommendation is 800 mg/day as the maximum dose.

Points to Remember

1. When administering eyedrops, avoid dropping them directly on the sensitive central cornea. Instead, release the drops into the lower conjunctival fornix.
2. Never give a patient a prescription for a topical anesthetic (or a sample, either).
3. Never use atropine or scopolamine to dilate the pupil for a fundus examination.

4. Never use or prescribe a topical ocular corticosteroid unless you have a precise diagnosis for which the drug is specifically indicated. You must be prepared to monitor the patient for serious side effects, such as glaucoma or cataract.

Sample Problems

1. A busy student comes to you during exam week because she is experiencing severe headaches. As part of a complete physical, you perform a basic eye examination. During ophthalmoscopy, you cannot fully see the optic disc because the patient's pupil is very small. You find no contraindications to dilating the pupil so you decide to do so to facilitate ophthalmoscopy. Your patient is brown-eyed, 20 years old, and has no other health complaint. Which of the following drugs would you select to dilate the pupils?

   a. Phenylephrine hydrochloride 0.12%
   b. Phenylephrine hydrochloride 2.5%
   c. Phenylephrine hydrochloride 10%
   d. Atropine sulfate 1%
   e. Tropicamide plus phenylephrine hydrochloride 2.5%

   Answer: e. The patient is experiencing severe headaches. A potential source of these headaches is increased intracranial pressure due to brain tumor, with resultant papilledema. Therefore, it is important to see the optic disc clearly to examine for these findings. Phenylephrine hydrochloride 2.5% may not be effective when used alone as a mydriatic in a brown-eyed patient. Atropine sulfate 1% is never used for simple pupillary dilation because its effects may last 1 to 2 weeks. The 0.12% solution of phenylephrine is the strength found in many over-the-counter ocular decongestants and will dilate the pupil minimally. The 10% solution is not the preferred concentration because it may be associated with serious systemic side effects in certain individuals. A combination of tropicamide with phenylephrine 2.5% usually provides excellent pupillary dilation with a relatively short duration of action and minimal systemic risk.

2. A man who has recently moved to the area is referred to you by a friend. He reports feeling especially tired lately, becoming fatigued after only moderate activity. He is also concerned about his vision; everything seems "dingy" or "yellow" to him. He's not sure when this visual symptom started. The patient has a history of heart disease, for which he takes cardiac medications. Examination reveals no health problems, other than his heart condition, which appears stable. How would you treat this patient? Should you refer him to an ophthalmologist at this time?

   Answer: Symptoms of blurred vision or abnormally colored vision occur with digitalis intoxication. Fatigue and weakness are also characteristic. Usually, such symptoms occur only with overdosage and resolve with reduction of dosage or discontinuation of the drug. Because no other health problems exist, it is reasonable to attribute his symptoms to digitalis intoxication. The step to take in this case is to measure the digitalis level in the blood and, if elevated, reduce the dose of digitalis. The patient should be monitored until the visual symptoms and fatigue are eliminated. Referral to an ophthalmologist is not necessary if the visual symptoms resolve.

3. A 25-year-old man makes an appointment to see you for complaints of difficulty breathing that developed after an injury. While playing basketball, he was knocked to the floor and struck his head. He went to the emergency room, where the only problem noted was a small hyphema in the right eye. He was seen by an ophthalmologist, who subsequently saw the patient for a return visit and instituted a pressure drop in the injured eye. The next day he developed shortness of breath and wheezing, and he asked to see you as he feared he may also have injured his chest when he fell. He thinks his parents told him he once had a brief episode of asthmatic bronchitis as a child, but he had previously felt this was not worth mentioning, as the condition required no chronic followup or therapy. What other history might be helpful for you in evaluating this patient's current symptoms? Would consultation with the ophthalmologist be necessary?

Answer: The onset of symptoms suggestive of asthma or other obstructive airway disease after institution of an ocular anti-hypertensive drop should make the clinician highly suspicious that the patient has been placed on a topical beta-blocker. Systemic absorption of either selective or nonselective drops in this class may be sufficient to cause significant contraction of bronchial smooth muscle, especially in asthmatics. The ophthalmologist should be contacted to determine the exact ocular medication regime and to inform him or her about the development of the side effects. The topical beta-blocker should be discontinued immediately, but because the intraocular pressure could subsequently rise to a dangerous level, the ophthalmologist should be consulted to determine if further ocular assessment or alternative drop therapy is advised.

Annotated Resources

Elson WL, Fraunfelder FT, Fills JN, et al: Adverse respiratory and cardiovascular events attributed to timolol ophthalmic solution, 1978–1985. *Am J Ophthalmol* 1986;102:606–611. A good general overview of various ocular and systemic complications associated with Timoptic.

Fraunfelder FT, Roy FH, eds: *Current Ocular Therapy 4*. Philadelphia: WB Saunders Co; 1995. An extensive text written by approximately 70 contributing authors and edited by two experienced ophthalmologists. Coverage is wide and fairly detailed, with a good emphasis on drug complications.

Grant WM, Schuman JS: *Toxicology of the Eye.* 4th ed. Springfield, IL: Charles C Thomas; 1993. Another encyclopedic treatment. A prodigious and scholarly work, carefully documenting ocular and neuro-ocular side effects of numerous chemicals and drugs.

Hardman JG: *Goodman and Gilman's The Pharmacologic Basis of Therapeutics.* 9th ed. New York: Pergamon Press; 1996. One of the best basic science textbooks on drugs. Serves as an encyclopedic reference on drugs in general.

Mauger TF: *Havener's Ocular Pharmacology.* 6th ed. St Louis: CV Mosby Co; 1994. A readily comprehended book with good emphasis on side effects and complications.

McMahan CD, Shaffer RN, Hoskins HD, et al: Adverse effects experienced by patients taking timolol. *Am J Ophthalmol* 1979;88:736–738. A good general reference regarding potential side effects of Timoptic, including a specific case report of a patient similar to that in Sample Problem 3 in this chapter.

Physicians' Desk Reference for Ophthalmology. Oradell, NJ: Medical Economics Co; updated annually. A slim volume distilling from the encyclopedic *PDR* those drugs used by ophthalmologists. As in the parent volume, the text of the package insert for each drug is reproduced. Supplementary charts, tables, and flow charts of use to clinicians are included. Besides sections on ophthalmic lenses and low vision, the book contains a reprint of the American Medical Association's *Guide to the Evaluation of Permanent Visual Impairment.*

Schoene RB, Martin TR, Charan NB, et al: Timolol-induced bronchospasm in asthmatic bronchitis. *JAMA* 1981;245:1460–1461.

Trobe JD: *The Physician's Guide to Eye Care.* San Francisco: American Academy of Ophthalmology; 1993. Chapters 6 and 7 deal respectively with common ocular medications and with ocular side effects of systemic drugs.

Index

Note: Page numbers in *italics* indicate illustrations; tables are indicated by *t*.

Note: Page numbers in *italics* indicate illustrations; tables are indicated by *t*.

Note: Page numbers in *italics* indicate illustrations; tables are indicated by *t*.

Note: Page numbers in *italics* indicate illustrations; tables are indicated by *t*.

D

Note: Page numbers in *italics* indicate illustrations; tables are indicated by *t*.

Note: Page numbers in *italics* indicate illustrations; tables are indicated by *t*.

Note: Page numbers in *italics* indicate illustrations; tables are indicated by *t*.

Note: Page numbers in *italics* indicate illustrations; tables are indicated by *t*.

Note: Page numbers in *italics* indicate illustrations; tables are indicated by *t.*

Note: Page numbers in *italics* indicate illustrations; tables are indicated by *t*.

Note: Page numbers in *italics* indicate illustrations; tables are indicated by *t*.

Note: Page numbers in *italics* indicate illustrations; tables are indicated by *t*.

Note: Page numbers in *italics* indicate illustrations; tables are indicated by *t*.

Note: Page numbers in *italics* indicate illustrations; tables are indicated by *t*.

Note: Page numbers in *italics* indicate illustrations; tables are indicated by *t.*

Note: Page numbers in *italics* indicate illustrations; tables are indicated by *t*.